CLINICAL PRACTICE OF HYPNOTHERAPY

The Guilford Clinical and Experimental Hypnosis Series
Michael J. Diamond and Helen M. Pettinati, Editors

CLINICAL PRACTICE OF HYPNOTHERAPY
M. Erik Wright with Beatrice A. Wright

In Preparation

HYPNOSIS, WILL, AND MEMORY: A PSYCHOLEGAL HISTORY
Jean-Roch Laurence and Campbell Perry

HYPNOSIS AND MEMORY
Helen M. Pettinati, Editor

CLINICAL PRACTICE OF HYPNOTHERAPY

M. Erik Wright, MD, PhD
with
Beatrice A. Wright, PhD

Foreword by Robert E. Pearson, MD

THE GUILFORD PRESS
New York   London

© 1987 The Guilford Press
A Division of Guilford Publications, Inc.
200 Park Avenue South, New York, N.Y. 10003

Printed in the United States of America

Last digit is print number: 9   8   7   6   5   4   3   2   1

Library of Congress Cataloging-in-Publication Data

Wright, M. Erik.
    Clinical practice of hypnotherapy

    (The Guilford clinical and experimental hypnosis
    series)
    Includes bibliographies and index.
    1. Hypnotism—Therapeutic use. 2. Psychotherapy.
I. Wright, Beatrice Ann Posner
II. Title. [DNLM: 1. Hypnosis—methods.   WM 415 W952h]
RC495.W75 1987   616.89′162   86-18473
ISBN 0-89862-337-5

To our enhanced family

Foreword

In musing over what I want said in this foreword, I am reminded of a story Abraham Lincoln told that ends with a man who was being tarred and feathered saying "If it weren't for the honor of it all, I'd rather be somewhere else." In this case that thought is very nicely balanced by another Lincoln statement—"I must admit that I do have the taste of it in my mouth."

Thinking about Erik Wright brings to mind so many words. Gentle. Friend. Loving. Quiet. Scholarly. Respectful. Honest. Open. Caring. Giving. Teacher. Thoughtful. Concerned. And many others like those, in many permutations and combinations.

To misquote Will Rogers, I never met a person who didn't like Erik. If there has been such, I'm content that we haven't met. On the other hand, as an inquisitive therapist, it might be clinically interesting to interview that person. But only once, thank you.

Obviously I believe that he was a remarkable person. But what else can you expect from someone who was chosen to write this from among so many others who could have been selected?

Erik received his first academic degree the year in which he had his 19th birthday. Degrees, honors, publications, and other facts fill many pages of his curriculum vitae, but they cannot tell what he was really like. This book describes the more important aspects of Erik very well.

It has been five-and-a-half years since he died, but it still feels as if he has just been out of touch for a while—perhaps on a sabbatical. And now that feeling is strongly reinforced; in a very real way he *is* back! The book he had been writing at the time of his death has been finished by his darling Beatrice. I cannot tell what is his and what is hers, nor do I wish to, but I can hear him clearly throughout the book.

Few therapists have been as committed as Erik was to searching for the essence of how to help people change, a commitment to explore and refine the techniques of psychotherapy. He was a devoted and tireless teacher. It was almost impossible to engage in any encounter with him, seemingly even the most casual of conversations, without having effortlessly acquired some new bit of knowledge or insight.

I believe that this is and will continue to be a significant book on the subject, useful to a large and varied audience. Even if the reader never has used, is not now using, or even never intends to use hypnosis as an adjunct to his or her practice (though that last is somewhat difficult to imagine if the book is read thoroughly), there is much to be learned here. Much about "ordinary" psychotherapy and much about human relationships as Erik saw and understood them. If I were still training therapists they would read this book early in the program. It would be of great help in orienting them to what I believe to be an essential aspect of the therapist–client relationship—*two-way respect and trust.*

The explanation of his principle of psychotherapy called comanagement (and I do believe that it was so characteristic of Erik's thinking that it can safely be called his) is of great value. All therapists of whatever orientation and experience will do very well to ponder those pages. If many prospective clients read and believed them there would be a real revolution in the management of psychological and physical problems.

Erik Wright's orientation was eclectic in the best positive sense of that word. These are the ideas that he found to be true for him. One of my teachers, John Dorsey, MD, told us over and over that we shouldn't believe anything he said just because he said it, that we would have to try out his ideas to see whether or not they were true for each of us, that to test them we would have to look within ourselves, and *that* would be the hardest work we would ever do. Erik had looked deeply within himself, found what was true for him, and then, fortunately for many of us, gently shared those ideas with those who would listen.

This book is not "The Compleat Hypnotherapist," nor was it intended to be. More could be said about many of the problems discussed, but what is there is almost all pure gold.

So please sit back, relax, let go of all the muscle tension that you don't need right now, let go of all of the mental stress that you don't need right now, find yourself reading easily and effortlessly, and l–i–s–t–e–n.

You will be well rewarded.

Robert E. Pearson, MD
November 1986

Preface

M. Erik Wright died on May 11, 1981. The deep sense of loss, affection, and appreciation felt by hundreds of persons throughout the country was expressed so well by one friend that I would like to reproduce it here:

"Erik added to the sum of human joy and fulfillment. If everyone to whom he did some loving service were to bring a blossom to his grave, he would sleep forever beneath a wilderness of flowers."

At the time of his death, Erik was immersed in a book-length manuscript on hypnotherapy. There never was any doubt in my mind that I would be the one who would continue the work of preparing the book for publication. As a psychologist familiar with the field of hypnosis, and as the wife of the author for many years, I felt that I was in a unique position to undertake the editing task in a way that would retain the meaning of what Erik had written, as well as capture the essence of the values and principles that guided him in helping people move toward constructive change.

As I proceeded with the task, inevitable problems arose. A voluminous amount of writing had to be reviewed. Some of it had been separated into chapters designated for the hypnotherapy book. Other writings were included in the material for a particular graduate course or workshop, and still others were filed under subject areas, such as smoking or sexual dysfunction. Fortunately, Erik had prepared a list of chapter headings, topics, and ideas to be encompassed by the book which helped guide the selection and integration of the material into a cohesive manuscript. Unfortunately, I was not able to find a way to integrate all of the important ideas. Also, in the process of editing and organizing the material into a book, it sometimes became necessary to clarify what had been written and to prepare transitions between separate sections. I only hope that the final manuscript has done justice to the richness of Erik's thinking.

References posed a different problem. Although the drafts with which I was working indicated places for references, I was unable to locate a reference file. Therefore, only those references for which I was able to obtain a complete citation are included. Actually, although it is clear that Erik benefited greatly from the work of others, the lack of references is not a serious omission, for the book so clearly represents the author's own philosophy and distinctive approach that it could very easily have been entitled "The Hypnotherapy of M. Erik Wright." Still, I apologize to those who would have been recognized had the author been able to complete the book.

The book is intended for professionals and advanced students in the fields of medicine, psychology, and social work. An overview of its organization is presented in the Table of Contents and at the end of the first chapter. The reader is cautioned that it will be necessary to carefully study the chapters of Parts I and II in order to appreciate the potential usefulness of various hypnotherapeutic approaches as they are applied and illustrated, sometimes but briefly, with respect to the special clinical problems discussed in Part III.

A word about the protocols. Most of the examples illustrating client–therapist interactions are from tape-recorded transcriptions of actual cases, with editorial modification as needed for purposes of clarification, preservation of anonymity, or brevity. I know that Erik would want me to express his profound appreciation to each one of his clients (patients) for the mutual affection and regard that developed between them and for the learning and growth that took place as a result of the therapeutic relationship.

To those with whom he worked so closely and from whom he learned so much in the American Society of Clinical Hypnosis and the Society for Clinical and Experimental Hypnosis, Erik would wish me to express what they must already know, namely, how deeply he valued the professional stimulation and bond of friendship. I would list their names were it not for the fear of important omissions. I am grateful for knowing at least some of them and for the support these friends offered me during the difficult time following Erik's death.

*   *   *

M. Erik Wright, MD, PhD, was Professor of Psychology and Psychiatry at The University of Kansas for 30 years and served there as Director of the Graduate Training Program in Clinical Psychology for 23 years. He received national recognition in the fields of hypnotherapy, psychotherapy, and sex therapy, and was widely sought as a workshop leader and teacher in these fields.

The M. Erik Wright Distinguished Professorship in Clinical Psychology has been established at The University of Kansas. I am ever grateful to the University and to the Department of Psychology for honoring Erik in this way. It was especially through the devoted efforts of C. Richard Snyder, Director of the Graduate Training Program in Clinical Psychology at the University, that the necessary funding in partial support of the Professorship was raised. My heart-felt thanks go to Dr. Snyder, as well as an abiding affection and esteem.

Many hundreds of students, colleagues, and friends donated to the Professorship. I would like them to know that not only was their financial support appreciated, but also their wish to preserve the spirit and contributions of the life and work of M. Erik Wright.

Beatrice A. Wright, PhD
April 1986

Contents

PART II. HYPNOTHERAPEUTIC APPROACHES

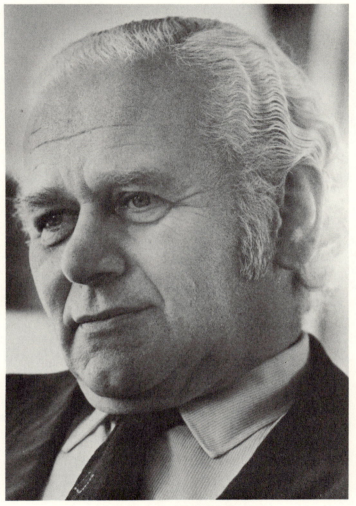

M. ERIK WRIGHT
(photograph taken in 1979)

CLINICAL PRACTICE OF HYPNOTHERAPY

I

INTRODUCTORY CONCEPTS AND GUIDELINES

Hypnotherapy and Psychotherapy

Hypnotherapy is the therapeutic use of the hypnotic state of consciousness as *part* of a psychotherapeutic intervention in order to enhance the effectiveness of the client's utilization of psychotherapy. It does not presume to provide a theoretical system that deals with the nature of personality or behavior, out of which would evolve the strategies for change derived from that system. That is the goal and the task of the individual systems of psychotherapy.

THE PLACE OF HYPNOTHERAPY IN PSYCHOTHERAPY

The conditions associated with the induction of hypnosis and the phenomenology of the hypnotic state itself are compatible with the goals and orientation of most systems of psychotherapy: namely, the development of a psychological climate in which the client can begin to consider or strengthen the possibility of change; the creation of an environment where the experience of change can be vicariously tried out in imagination and fantasy; and the fostering of trust between client and therapist that sustains continuing progress and behavior change in real life. How the hypnotic state of consciousness is used in therapy, however, depends upon the clinician's psychotherapeutic orientation, the clinician's personality, the client's problem and personality, and the client's general situation. This holds with respect to preferred methods of trance induction and the selection of experiences during the hypnotic state that will help the client progress toward the therapeutic goals.

Hypnotherapy and Behavior Therapy

Although hypnotherapy is often classified among the behavior therapies, the point should be stressed that hypnosis as a tool can be effectively used with insight-oriented as well as behavior-oriented therapies. The term "behavior" needs clarification. In its broader sense, behavior includes such internal events as perceptions, affects, beliefs, and attitudes, as well as events observable by others (namely, what the person says and does). In its narrower sense, behavior refers to the latter—that is, to overt behavior. Although the emphasis placed on directly altering overt behavior varies with the therapeutic approach, change in overt behavior receives attention, along with probing for understanding, as an intermixed part of psychotherapy in general. Where client understanding is not sought as part of the process, the therapeutic approach is not grouped among the *psychotherapies*.

In subsequent chapters, examples are presented in which hypnosis is used to gain insight and understanding, as well as to modify behavior directly, including a focus on symptom removal (or symptom substitution in the case of a less disturbing alternative).

The Psychotherapeutic Premise

The fundamental premise of all psychotherapy is that some kinds of human problems can be alleviated by using language to communicate ideas and feelings. Language encompasses both verbal and nonverbal communication through the use of sounds, gestures, or signs that have symbolic meaning. Thus, when communication can be established between the troubled person and a chosen other or others, or with oneself, it becomes possible for a process to begin that is called "psychological healing."

The chosen other may or may not be a professional therapist. It may be a peer counselor or friend, a parent or teacher. Furthermore, self-reflection, in which the person attends to different aspects of his or her self and life, also involves psychological messages that can be helpful. Actually, most psychological healing occurs through self-reflection. It is when problems remain despite this form of self-help that the person turns to others.

Although there are many psychotherapies varying in important aspects of theory and practice, they agree that language can be used as a medium for effecting change in thoughts and feelings, attitudes and values, habits and behavior, and physiological states. In the case of physical symptoms, language can sustain or evoke bodily experiences that occurred in the past. Long after a disturbing biological event (e.g., pain) or psychological event (e.g., rejection) with its physical repercussions has subsided, the memory of the event may continue to maintain body mobilization to deal with the stress. The mobilization of the body to meet the original stress may persist to a degree that interferes with the recovery process or may become easily triggered under ordinarily innocuous circumstances.

Verbal language and other symbols are a vehicle for reinstating body states in general. States of excitement (as in the case of pleasure and anticipation), states of stress (as in the case of frustration and failure), and states of calmness (as in the case of restfulness and serenity) can be invoked by recalling events and conditions that gave rise to them in the past. Various psychotherapies make use of language to reach into past memories and images—sometimes to evoke particular body states for catharsis or other purposes; sometimes to enable the person to reinterpret past events; and sometimes to make use of past memories and images in dealing with current problems and circumstances. Whatever the case, the particular content and form of the language used in hypnotherapy is guided by the therapist's psychotherapeutic orientation.

Suitability of Different Psychotherapeutic Approaches

All psychotherapeutic approaches have a system of beliefs about the nature and characteristics of human personality, the significant variables affecting human functioning, and the ways in which behavior can best be changed. These belief systems may be vaguely or more systematically defined, and may be closely or loosely related to the psychotherapeutic strategies and procedures used to help individuals move toward improving their lives. In the literature, the commonly identified psychotherapies are sometimes classified according to such terms as "psychoanalytically oriented," "client-centered," "existential," "humanistic" and "behavior-oriented" therapy.

The belief systems or theories elaborate notions of personality development and the origins of emotional problems in more or less detail. From these notions, the goals of therapy, the nature of the desired relationship between therapist and client, and specialized strategies or procedures to bring about desired change emerge. Some theories emphasize, as an overarching goal, the need to effect fundamental change in the client's personality, whereas others are more concerned with enabling the client to function more adequately within the existing basic personality. Some theories focus on the past and others on the present. Some theories are directed toward uncovering unconscious motives and repressed memories, whereas others are concerned with more conscious levels of awareness. Some theories consider the transference relationship between client and therapist as essential, whereas others hold that it is more fruitful to view the relationship on a here-and-now reality basis. Some theories require the therapist to be at the helm in directing the therapeutic action; others affirm a more nondirective therapist role. Some theories stress sociocultural–environmental factors; others give little weight to these circumstances. And so forth. As for specialized procedures, a rich panoply has emerged from the variety of theories concerning personality development and behavior change. A sample includes free association, reflection of feelings, dream interpretation, group and family therapy, psychodrama, contingencies of reinforcement, biofeedback, and hypnosis.

The suffix "-therapy" in the word "psychotherapy" should be given some thought so as to avoid the gratuitous assumption that the person coming for help has some form of pathology or disease to be cured by the clinician. Alternative terms, such as "psycho-education," "psycho-conversion," "psycho-counseling," "psycho-prayer," or "psycho-debate," more aptly describe the type of client–therapist interaction, goals, and philosophy of one or another "psycho-therapy."

The effectiveness of different psychotherapeutic approaches in alleviating distress has been difficult to assess for many reasons. One reason is that the term "psychotherapeutic approach" itself, as commonly used, has different referents. Sometimes it refers to the underlying theory of personality and behavior change on which it is based; sometimes to the nature of the therapist–client relationship; sometimes to particular short- or long-range goals; sometimes to specific procedures; and sometimes to all of these in imprecisely defined combinations. Additionally, the complexities of the psychosocial characteristics of the client and therapist—including their varied sociocultural backgrounds and values, the unique aspects of the client's difficulties and situation, and the skill level that the therapist brings to a given therapeutic approach—make understandable the impossibility of evaluating outcome effectiveness by simply classifying clients' problems and types of psychotherapy, establishing outcome criteria, and evaluating the results. Fortunately, a large body of research has tended to affirm the potential effectiveness of psychotherapy in general. It has clarified some of the basic conceptual and methodological issues involved in outcome research and has revealed important characteristics common to most schools of psychotherapy.

The clinician is obliged to work with the client even without full assurance as to how best to proceed. Actually, the different systems of psychotherapy, nomenclature notwithstanding, often significantly overlap in their aims and methods so that it is possible to view the collective clinical experience as offering several potentially promising interventions that can be made compatible with the clinician's orientation. If one strategy or tactic proves wanting, others can be sought and adapted.

Therapists of different persuasions have applied hypnosis, as a special state of consciousness, in divergent ways to facilitate the following processes:

1. *Cognitive restructuring.* By exploring feelings, experiences, and knowledge of events related to present fears and reactions, the client is helped to alter perceptions of the self, of others, and of situations. Such re-evaluation allows new ways of coping and interacting to become viable possibilities.

2. *Abreaction, catharsis, desensitization.* Through the releasing of feelings in a benign situation, fears and anger become dissipated. This release, plus the support and emergence of hidden positive aspects of relived experiences, make it easier to reframe the meaning and significance of past and present situations.

3. *Symptom modification.* Through relaxation, pain and obsessional fears are reduced or eliminated, permitting the person to gain greater control over their occurrence in real life.

4. *Education and rehabilitation.* Practicing altered modes of thinking, feeling, and imaged behavior under hypnosis reinforces the new learnings and their application to everyday life situations.

It is essential to reaffirm the basic principle that hypnosis is not a system of psychotherapy, or a theory of personality, or a philosophy of treatment. The hypnotic trance is a state of consciousness introduced to help expedite psychotherapeutic activity. It should also be recognized that the inappropriate use of hypnotic trance may interfere with the therapeutic process.

The psychological treatment of any problem reflects the ideas or theory that the psychotherapist believes best defines the nature of the problem, its etiology, its maintenance, and the course of action likely to bring about improvement. Thus, when the therapist is evaluating the use of hypnotic trance in the treatment of particular problems, two separate questions are involved. The most important question is whether the psychotherapeutic system invoked has helped the particular client progress toward desired goals. The second question is whether the use of hypnotic trance as part of that system has been helpful or not. The central issue about the use of hypnotic trance, therefore, is its role vis-à-vis facilitating the broader psychotherapeutic process and not the question of whether hypnotic trance, regarded in a psychotherapeutic vacuum, has been an effective treatment by itself. Simply put, the way hypnosis is applied is always implicitly or explicitly tied to the therapist's philosophical and psychological belief system or theory concerning human development, the conditions that facilitate or impede growth, and the ways in which to help the client bring about constructive change.

Further elucidation of the potential utilization of clinical hypnosis within the main currently practiced systems of psychotherapy is beyond the scope of the present work. Instead, later chapters demonstrate a selection of hypnotherapeutic procedures that can usefully be adapted to fit a variety of psychotherapeutic approaches.[1]

AUTHOR'S APPROACH AND THE BASIC PRINCIPLE OF COMANAGEMENT

I should like to orient the reader briefly to my own psychotherapeutic approach. Generally, it would be regarded as an eclectic approach in which the client's thoughts, feelings, and overt behavior become the focus of interpretation, reflection, suggestion, and differential reinforcement at various times during the course of psychotherapy. Current problems of living guide the examination of present viewpoints and feelings, past memories and experiences, and future hopes and expectations, in order to further the understanding of problems and issues. The client tries out new coping strategies to effect change in the self, in relationships with others, and in the situation. Fundamental is a respect for the client, a respect that includes an appreciation of the client's struggles and potential for growth.

1. The reader may be interested in the book, *Case Studies in Hypnotherapy*, edited by E. T. Dowd and J. M. Healy (New York: Guilford Press, 1986). The cases were solicited from therapists with varying theoretical orientations.

Perhaps my approach is best captured within a field-dynamic framework that conceives of psychotherapy as an educational opportunity—a learning experience in which old cognitions are modified, now affective associaions formed, new behaviors made possible, and the life space restructured. Since reality factors in the environment significantly affect possibilities for change, they are seriously taken into account.

Throughout the therapeutic process, one of the main principles guiding my relationship with the client is the principle of comanagement. "Comanagement" conveys the idea of mutually agreed-upon procedures relating to the therapeutic interaction. It therefore requires that the client be well informed of the nature of hypnosis. It suggests that the client be encouraged to contribute ideas about how to bring about constructive change. It implies that clarification of interpretations and suggestions is a natural part of the interaction. It means that the right of the client to become actively engaged in guiding the therapeutic course and in rejecting unacceptable suggestions is respected.

The question of the use of the terms "client" and "patient" is germane to the comanagement principle. Unfortunately, the term "patient" carries surplus meaning that often, if not typically, jars with the comanagement concept. It frequently connotes the "sick role," a role of dependency and hierarchy in which the superior knowledge of the doctor requires that the patient cooperate with prescribed procedures. This is unfortunate because not all doctor-patient relationships are defined by this uni-directional line of command. The comanagement principle, on the other hand, clearly regards the person seeking help as a full-fledged partner, with decision-making responsibilities concerning the therapeutic process. Also, the idea of "patient" generally applies to a person who is physically ill or in a hospital, whereas "client" is more inclusive in its application. It is for these reasons that the term "client" is used throughout the present volume, although some therapists are accustomed to, and might prefer, the alternative term. I too have referred to "patients" in other writings.

The principle of comanagement supports the need of the client to gain a sense of control over important aspects of his or her life. Changes in the manner of experiencing and expressing the self, as well as changes in the client's situation and relationships with others, are sought. The client comes to the therapist seeking help because of loss of control over events that threaten the client's sense of well-being. The client has tried out a repertory of coping strategies, but has not significantly diminished the distress. Often the distress seems to be on the increase, and the client may actually experience loss of control over his or her life. The therapist is sought because of an anticipated potential for expanding the client's control over events and reducing stress.

Yet, there may be ambivalence about regaining control, for frequently special advantages accrue to the "sick" or "incapacitated" role. There may also be ambivalence about the therapist, based on fear that the therapist's intervention may impair the already weakened sense of control. The therapist accepts the client's need for increasing the capacity to control stressful events in his or her life while recognizing likely ambivalence in this regard. The comanagement principle, by underscoring the *leadership* of both client *and* therapist in the therapeutic effort, fits well with the client's need to become a more effective agent in influencing his or her life, as well as with any ambivalence about doing so.

Because it is important to establish the client's role from the start as one who is actively involved in participating and influencing the psychotherapeutic process, assessment or diagnostic procedures are not regarded as precursors to treatment. Instead, assessment is viewed as part of the psychotherapeutic process itself. The comanagement principle suggests, therefore, that the client is encouraged to become actively involved in determining both the utilization and evaluation of assessment indicators.

As will be observed later, it is because of the comanagement principle that I so frequently seek permission from the client to proceed in one way or another. It is also because of this principle that I offer the client the opportunity to record therapy sessions on tape and to utilize hypnotic procedures for self-improvement at home. Listening to the tapes and practicing at home encourage the comanagement role. They also reinforce new learning and facilitate the discovery of new insights.

PLAN OF THE BOOK

The present volume is divided into three parts. Part I, consisting of three chapters, sets the stage for the use of hypnosis as an aid in the psychotherapy of actual life problems. It deals with such introductory topics as the relationship between hynotherapy, psychotherapy, and behavior therapy; my own orientation; the nature of the trance state of consciousness; conditions facilitating the trance experience; the hypnotherapy of language usage; nonverbal ways of signaling thoughts and feelings; and methods of helping the client experience trance at different levels.

The five chapters of Part II describe and provide examples of a variety of specific hypnotherapeutic procedures useful in treatment, such as guided imagery, projective techniques, and dissociation. They were selected as prototypes and also as being suggestive of other procedures that can become part of an expanding repertoire.

Part III focuses on different clinical problems, with separate chapters devoted to pain, smoking, overeating, sexual dysfunction, sleep disturbances, and crisis intervention. The historical and cultural context, biological aspects, and current theories are brought to bear in understanding the nature of these problems. Hynotherapeutic applications are indicated and brief examples provided, with the expectation that the reader will be able to elaborate the examples on the basis of the procedures described earlier in considerably greater detail.

Preparing for the Trance Experience

HYPNOTIC-LIKE EXPERIENCES IN EVERYDAY LIFE

It is important to remember that a number of characteristics of the hypnotic state are commonly experienced in everyday living. Consider the influence of suggestion. As an example, certain tastes in foods, soap, and fashion are acquired because of suggestions in the advertising media. Those suggestions that we accept become so much a part of ourselves that we forget their original source. Yet, clearly, accepting a suggestion is not an automatic response. We somehow exercise a selective choice among the great variety of suggestions before us. Similarly, in the case of hypnotherapy, there is not an automatic acceptance of all suggestions. However, the therapist attempts to create the conditions that will permit an optimal consideration of the therapeutic suggestion—and that, in a sense, is why the hypnotic state has such positive therapeutic potential.

Everyday life also makes us acquainted with many situations in which we withdraw from the immediate reality. Thus, a boring lecture, a late staff meeting, or a long wait under the hair dryer will find us "drifting away" into ourselves with eyes open. This drifting away can occur even when we need to attend to our surroundings. A case in point is becoming immersed in our own thoughts while driving along a familiar route. Remaining unconsciously alert, we arrive safely at the destination, and are startled to discover that we have no recollection of having traversed the course. A curious bypass of the usual audiovisual stimuli from consciousness has taken place. Then, when the particular event is over, it does not feel as if we have been asleep, but only withdrawn into a special personal space.

Yet another type of general withdrawal can occur while we are deeply concentrating on an ongoing activity. Most of us have had the experience of becoming so involved with a book or TV program that we remain oblivious of someone entering the room. Sometimes we do not even notice the discomfort of the aborted blood supply to a foot tucked underneath ourselves. Only when the involvement is interrupted do we become aware of a sharp inflow of stimuli from both the internal and external environment, which clearly informs us that we have been "someplace else" psychologically for a time.

Everyday life also teaches us that ideas, words, and other symbols are intimately coordinated with sensory awareness and muscle tone. We need only to see the roller coaster going down the steep incline in the Cinerama movie to have a tightening of our stomach muscles, or to hear someone describe a favorite dish until we almost taste and smell it. We have also learned that when we are in environments where distracting stimuli are reduced (e.g., the movies, resting, daydreaming, sleeping), then our thoughts and fantasies may acquire added vividness and experiential intensity.

It is important to state again that almost all phenomena elicited during hypnosis can also occur in the "waking state." To respond to suggestions, to daydream, to block recall, and to become so involved in an ongoing activity as to exclude pain and fatigue are experiences available to people both in the "waking state" and in the "hypnotic state" under appropriate conditions. The significant point with respect to therapy is that, by teaching the client to enter the state of hypnosis, it is possible to help the client re-experience past events and envision new possibilities in such a manner as to contribute to achieving the therapeutic goals toward which he or she is striving.

CLARIFYING COMMON MISCONCEPTIONS

Two general, not mutually exclusive circumstances are associated with the decision to use hypnotherapeutic procedures with a given client. In the first case, the client is self-referred or referred by another person to a therapist with known interest and competence in hypnosis. The client may then feel, "Everything else has been tried and found wanting; this is my last hope." Although this attitude may strengthen the client's motivation for change, it also may intensify his or her fear of failure and apprehension about the treatment. In the second case, the client is not referred for hypnosis, but the therapist, preferably in consultation with the client, reaches the conclusion that hypnosis could be helpful. In either case, it is generally necessary to clarify misconceptions about the nature of hypnosis with the client, for misconceptions about hypnosis are widespread. Magical thinking, exaggerated statements of hypnotic powers, and fears of being controlled are all part of the mythology.

A basic myth is the belief that the hypnotic state is one that has to be imposed upon the individual by another person, rather than a state in which the individual, guided by the hypnotist, places the self. A corollary to this belief is that the individual is unconscious during hypnosis. To remind all of us that this is not the case, and that consciousness remains even in deep states of hypnosis, such phrases as "the hypnotic state of consciousness" and "trance consciousness" appear throughout the present volume. Even where posthypnotic amnesia is an outcome, it is the client who has accepted the amnesia. Clients need to understand that the hypnotized person remains capable of higher mental processes, such as forming judgments, making decisions, and guiding his or her own behavior, although subconscious factors may also become more apparent.

A subtle variation of the theme that hypnosis is imposed on the person is the idea that being able to go into hypnosis is indicative of gullibility. An important distinction needs to be made in this connection. Gullibility is the lack of discriminatory and judgmental abilities. Clients need to be reassured that suggestibility, on the other hand, is regarded as a *capacity* to utilize a verbal or nonverbal concept after integrating it into one's functioning.

It is worth noting that sometimes the effectiveness of hypnosis may partly be due to fantasies about the capacity of the individual to be transformed when "hypnotized." The individual may desire to shift responsibility for his or her actions to the therapist and to behave in a way that would ordinarily be restrained in the nonhypnotic state. The myths associated with being controlled, however, may also be therapeutically disruptive, for clients usually have a normal ambivalence about psychotherapy (i.e., "Will it help matters, or will I be worse off than before?"). Anxiety over the possible use and misuse of hypnotic procedures is likely to increase resistance. That is why it is important to clarify misconceptions, not only initially, but throughout the course of therapy as questions arise.

The therapist's conception of hypnosis and the style of therapist–client interaction greatly influence the substance and manner of dealing with clients' myths about hypnosis. My preferred way of responding to the common concerns of clients is presented below. The reader will notice how my own psychotherapeutic orientation becomes integrated into the clarification process, especially with regard to (1) insuring the client's control and freedom of choice in the situation; (2) sharing knowledge with the client; (3) supporting the client's readiness for growth and capability of utilizing therapy constructively; and (4) respecting the client's judgment and decisions.

1. *"What if something should happen to you, Doctor, while I am in trance?"*

The explanation I offer follows these lines: "When you close your eyes and permit your mind and body to relax, your total level of tension and stress decreases. Even though you become quite indifferent to noises and all sorts of distractions both in your environment and in your own body, and even though your thoughts and images take you far away from the immediate scene here, you are and will remain *totally conscious at all times.* Your mind will remain active. You have it within you to terminate the trance at any time you may choose to decide that that is what you want to do. You may choose not to terminate the trance because what you are experiencing is helpful to you in your progress toward better functioning. At no time are you in any state resembling unconsciousness, even when all experience of pain may be blocked off. Thus, if I should suddenly leave, or collapse, you would be aware of the situation. You would arouse yourself, or if you wish, permit yourself to drift from the hypnotic state into a short period of sleep and then arouse yourself. In all cases you retain the capacity to arouse yourself when you decide that that is what you want to do."

2. *"What if I am not able to enter into hypnosis, not able to experience hypnosis?"*

"Everyone has already been in hypnosis as part of ordinary life experiences. As a fetus in your mother's womb, you have known what it is to be quieted when your mother walked and you were rocked back and forth in your amniotic fluid cradle. As a child and as an adult, you have already experienced becoming totally absorbed by a film or TV show so that you became quite unaware of your surroundings. People do differ in how quickly they learn to enter into hypnotic trance at will in specific situations. Even a state of relaxation can be therapeutically most helpful, and much can be accomplished with even very light states of hypnosis. To try too hard, or to worry about going into trance, may interfere with the natural process of relaxing and letting the feeling of inner security and peace develop. It may distract you from focusing upon the images that encourage detachment. As we become more comfortable with this new state of consciousness, we go further into hypnosis without effort. Moving into hypnotic trance becomes easier and more accessible."

3. *"Will I lose control over myself? Will you take control over me?"*

"When you experience the hypnotic state of consciousness, it is because you have the ability to concentrate, to let your muscles relax, to let yourself become detached from the bounds of the immediate situation. I am your guide, not your master. The trust that you give is what makes it possible for me, together with your guidance, to show you the way into trance and into utilizing hypnosis for treatment. You give your trust because you are searching for a way to improve your functioning in life. You retain the power to withdraw that trust and terminate the trance and even the relationship with me. At all times you will make use *only* of those suggestions that are therapeutically helpful to you and that fit with your basic values and beliefs."

4. *"Will I be unable to remember what happened during my hypnosis?"*

"Some people spontaneously close off their memory of what took place during the hypnotic trance when they arouse themselves. They have found that this makes it easier for them to work on some of their difficult problems. If they choose, they can be helped to remember everything that happened. Other people remember everything that went on during the hypnotic trance when they arouse themselves. Yet, they too can be taught to close off their memory until such time as they want to recall it. Whether a person remembers or closes off the memory of events in the hypnotic trance depends upon what the individual and therapist decide would be best for progress in treatment. Every person is capable of remembering everything that happens during the hypnotic state of consciousness, but he or she does not have to remember anything unless it is therapeutically useful."

Clients may raise many other questions, but these four, with some minor variations, are the ones I have most frequently encountered. The same client may raise the same question again, even though there has been adequate exploration the first time, but that is not unusual in any therapeutic interaction.

INTRODUCING THE CLIENT TO THE TRANCE STATE

Almost every client can experience some degree of hypnotic trance in a therapeutic relationship, and for many therapeutic purposes an extensive hypnotic involvement is not required. This section describes a number of introductory experiences with trance that may be helpful to the client, after a period of contact with the therapist in which preliminary assessment of the client's presenting problems has occurred and a decision has been reached by both the therapist and client to explore hypnotherapeutic methods that might be of value in the treatment plan.

Introductory trance experiences are helpful in several ways:

1. They introduce the client to the concept of "ideomotor behavior"—that is, to the impact of ideas and imagery upon body action even when there is no decision to respond in a particular way.
2. They provide the therapist with a rough impression of the client's relative guarding, tenseness, and imagery capability.
3. They provide a basis for the client to raise questions about misconceptions or concerns.

The four procedures described below may suggest other potentially useful approaches for the purpose of trance preparation. Not all procedures, clearly, are used with every client.

Arm-Weight Experience: Example of Procedure

The instructions are along the following lines:

"Please close your eyes and extend both arms as far forward as possible. On your stronger arm, imagine that a canvas bag has been slipped over the wrist, and visualize two heavy red bricks that have been put into the bag. Just let yourself feel the weight of these bricks in the bag. On your weaker hand, imagine a brilliantly colored balloon filled with helium tied to the wrist and tugging the arm upward so that it seems to want to float up higher and higher. Let the arm become lighter, and have the balloon pull this weaker arm up. In the meantime, the strong arm is being weighted down by the two red bricks in the canvas bag. Add two more bricks to the load and just feel the downward pull of all that weight. [The therapist should give these images a few more moments to develop their full effect.] Now open your eyes and notice what has happened. Isn't that interesting? Your weaker arm is floating comfortably up in the air, and the stronger one is pulled down quite a distance. Close your eyes again, shake your hands from the wrist to the shoulder, let the balloon go free, and discard the imaginary canvas bag and its bricks. Have both arms feel free of tension from the fingertips to the shoulders. Now let your eyes open. What do you make of this experience?"

A brief discussion follows as to why there was so much experienced tension in the stronger arm—how it felt so much more fatigued although both arms were exposed to the equal pull of gravitation downward. In this way, the power of ideomotor suggestion can be demonstrated.

Hand-Sculpture Experience: Example of Procedure

The instructions are roughly as follows:

"Please close your eyes. Intertwine the fingers of your right and left hands so that the palms are pressed tightly against each other, and raise the clenched hands over your head. As you press your two hands into each other, imagine that they are becoming blended together as if molded out of beautiful marble, all of a single piece. As the fingers press down onto the opposite hands, let them blend into the backs of these hands so that you can no longer distinguish which finger belongs to which hand. Everything is becoming a single beautiful unity exquisitely sculpted from a single piece of marble. Let yourself feel this unity, the oneness of the two hands. The more clearly and the more beautifully you visualize this piece of sculpture, the more oneness you feel in the hands; and if you try to move your hands apart, you will find resistance to their coming apart. Try taking them apart: The more you try, the more firmly the single beautiful sculpture prevails. Now stop trying and lower your hands to your lap. Let the sculpture dissolve and your two hands relax, become two again, and readily come apart, yet retain their feeling of being something beautiful. Now open your eyes. What do you think of this experience?"

In the discussion, I usually include the explanation that this particular maneuver is facilitated by both anatomy and neurophysiology, which make discrimination more difficult when the clasped hands are pressed against each other and elevated about the head. Imparting this information is an example of "giving knowledge away" unless thoughtful therapeutic judgment suggests otherwise. In addition, how imagery heightens the sense of inseparability of the hands is included in the discussion.

Umbrella Experience: Example of Procedure

Before proceeding, the therapist should ask the client whether he or she has had much experience with umbrellas. If the reply is affirmative, the therapist proceeds as follows:

"Please close your eyes. Imagine that you are walking in a light mist, and that you have a large black umbrella in your hand. In spite of the rain, you are feeling cheerful. Gradually let yourself feel a strong wind beginning to blow and lift up the umbrella. It amuses you to feel the wind lift the umbrella up higher and higher in the air. It is a real tugging up and down. The lift is so strong that it almost feels that it might be strong enough to lift you off the ground as your arm rises up in the air. Now let the umbrella go and watch the wind carry it away. It is all right to let go because it is an imaginary umbrella and you can always bring it back with just one thought. Let your arm relax to your side, and open your eyes."

The follow-up discussion often has the client talking about how vividly the lift was felt and how reluctant he or she was to release the umbrella until permission was given.

Sway Experience: Example of Procedure

If the client is considerably heavier than the therapist (e.g., 190 pounds vs. 110 pounds), then this procedure is not recommended.

The client is asked to stand up and the therapist stands behind him or her. If the client is a woman wearing high heels, the therapist asks whether she would feel comfortable standing in her stocking feet. The therapist then puts his or her hands gently on the shoulders of the client, gradually permitting them to come to rest so that the muscle tension of the shoulders can be felt beneath the hands of the therapist. The fingers are placed over the shoulder muscles, with the thumbs facing each other near the base of the neck to better experience the tension of the back muscles.

The instructions are as follows:

"Please put your heels together with your toes pointing forward. I am going to put my hands alongside your face and under your chin. Let me raise your head until you are watching the line where the ceiling and the wall meet. Keep your attention focused on that line.

"I shall let you know exactly what I plan to do before I do it so there will be nothing unexpected. I am going to place my hands alongside your shoulders and brace myself. Let me move you just a little bit over to the left. That's fine! Now, let me move you just a little bit over to the right. Very good.

"Now I am going to put my hands on your shoulders again. This time let me move you just a little bit forward. Very good! And now a little bit backward. Good. You have experienced me moving you to the left, to the right, forward, and backward with your eyes open. Now let me once again position your head [the therapist repeats the head-raising maneuver]. Focus on the same line but with your eyes closed.

"Now let me move you just a little bit toward the left. Fine! Now let me move you just a little bit right. Good! Now, let me move you just a little bit forward, and finally, let me move you just a little bit further backward. Very Good!

"Have you ever gone sailing? Do you enjoy the water? [If the answer is positive, the therapist proceeds; otherwise a different image is used—for example, the client has a heavy rucksack on his or her back and the therapist is pulling on the straps.]

"Now imagine yourself to be a mast with a universal joint at the ankles, and there is a beautiful sail attached to you. I have braced myself in back of you with my hands just a small distance back of your shoulders. Now let the warm pleasant breeze begin to blow against your chest and begin to move you backward. I am right behind you. Let that wind grow as strong as necessary to move that mast on its universal joint at the base."

The suggestions are maintained until a definite movement is observed. If a clear movement is not obtained, the suggestions are terminated, and the therapist can ask the client to describe how the experiences were experienced. If a clear movement is observed, the therapist may introduce yet another experience:

"That's fine. Now, I am going to place one hand on your shoulder, and with the other hand I am going to place this sturdy chair in back of you so that you can just feel the seat edge of the chair barely touching the back of your leg near the knees. I am going to brace myself and the chair. When you feel my hands at your elbows, your knees will gently unlock, and you will settle back very relaxed into the chair. Now, with your eyes closed and focused at the line where ceiling and wall meet, let this gentle, warm breeze begin to blow and become stronger and stronger. Fine, good. Now as you move backward, my hands are guiding you into the chair, and when you are in the chair, let the breeze, the sail, and everything related to this interesting image disappear and just let every muscle relax and enjoy the sensation of quietness.

"That's fine. Just let it continue for a few moments longer. Now very gently arouse yourself, let your normal tone return to your muscles, and let your eyes open. Tell me how you felt about each of these different experiences."

The sway experience serves the purpose of establishing trust between the client and the therapist. It also informs the therapist of whether the client shows ease of movement or is more guarded in accepting the therapeutic process. A possible discrepancy may be reflected between verbal assertions of trust and help seeking on the part of the client, and nonverbal communications of tension, apprehension, and the need to maintain vigilance.

In the sway procedure, the therapist repeats the phrase, "Let me move you." The request in that form is for permission and symbolizes "therapeutic movement" that goes beyond the immediate focus on body action. Some clients have reported at later stages in their therapy that they remembered this phrase and that it felt reassuring as well as hopeful. It is obviously difficult to assess the impact of any specific therapeutic interaction, yet it is reasonable to suppose that a statement such as this one, with its metaphoric implications, may have therapeutic significance for the client. The motivation to change, to allow oneself to be "moved," is an important part of what brings most clients into the therapeutic relationship.

GENERAL CONDITIONS FACILITATING TRANCE INDUCTION

Five general conditions that are often conducive to induction of hypnosis are briefly elaborated below. In the scientific sense, they are not considered "necessary and sufficient" since an individual can learn to go into the trance state of consciousness when one or more of the conditions are absent. Perhaps they should more properly be considered conditions that appear to facilitate induction.

Trust in Therapist

Trust in or rapport with the therapist provides support to the client and makes risk taking more tolerable, at least within the defined setting of the psychotherapeutic relationship. The sense of increased security, drawn in part from the therapist, seems to reflect itself in an increased readiness to enter trance. The client becomes more capable of setting aside those constraints that interfere with a freer use of fantasy and imagination as related to his or her inner experience. Trust in the therapist supports hope for the future, and thus a willingness to consider alternatives, options, and reinterpretations of ongoing emotional problems.

Reduction of Sensory Input

A quiet setting is recommended in which there is a reduction of distracting sounds, lights, and odors. A reasonably comfortable chair for the client, placed where kinesthetic stimuli are reduced, tends to be facilitating. Perhaps these conditions are favorable because they are associated with relaxation, reduction of vigilance, and a measure of enhanced security.

Fixation of Attention

The hypnotic state is not a passive bleaching out of cognitive function. On the contrary, various types of active fixation of attention, such as focusing on a light, a sound (metronome), a visual pattern, or an idea or fantasy, help to screen out distracting stimuli. The increased attention paid to the therapist's voice leads to a decreased intrusion of competing influences, thus allowing the therapist's suggestions to have a heightened impact.

Muscle Relaxation

Reduction in muscle tension with relaxation seems to facilitate the person's capability for letting the self experience the hypnotic state more fully. The decrease in "defensive posture" related to the lowered muscle tonus also seems to contribute to a decrease in psychological defensiveness as well. The fact that typically the client has closed his or her eyes provides a clear indication of some basic level of security vis-à-vis the therapist. This lowering of the stress level can be seen as a "psychological distancing" from the problems confronting the client. The more relaxed attitude is frequently associated with a decrease in the critical assessment of incoming stimuli, and this helps the client to lend the self to the hypnotic state of consciousness without challenging its reality.

Heightened Awareness of One's Inner Life

The focus upon some of the sensations from within one's body or upon fantasies or thoughts, further enhances the separation of the self from the broad spectrum of the external environment. The fantasies or thoughts, sensations or images, may be suggested by the therapist or chosen by the client, but focusing on the inner life and internal space makes possible a heightened responsiveness and openness toward certain kinds of thoughts and feelings that are usually less accessible to the client.

Many procedures are used in teaching the client how to enter the trance state of consciousness. Yet almost all methods seek to establish these five general conditions in order to support the induction experience.

THE HYPNOTHERAPY OF LANGUAGE USAGE

From the start, the induction procedure requires the therapist to offer suggestions as a way of guiding the person into the trance state. The *form* of a suggestion—not only its content—is important and will reflect the therapist's values and theory of change. The following 11 guidelines for the formulation of suggestions have considerable clinical usefulness. They are presented with the realization that some therapists may wish to modify or eliminate one or another according to their own proclivities.

Clarifying the Behavior Desired

In most, although not all, methods of induction training, the client needs to know what is expected in response to the therapist's instructions. Many clinical workers believe that the modified critical attitude that occurs during the trance state is accompanied by an increase in concrete thinking. Concrete thinking implies that the client becomes more literal in interpreting suggestions. It is therefore felt that suggestions should be presented in concrete terms, with as few equivocal words as possible. An action can be described in specific contexts instead of abstract generalities. When the changes explored during trance have been found productive, generalizing the behavior in terms of conceptualizing the issues can then be developed in the nonhypnotic state.

Respecting the Client's Language

This principle requires the therapist to respect the client's language and make use of it without parody or put-down. It also means that the therapist must use language understandable to the client and be careful about terms that are ambiguous or too abstract.

Formulating Suggestions Positively

A positive suggestion helps clients to think in terms of their goals and to organize their perceptions and actions accordingly, whereas a negative formulation provides no clue concerning the conditions conductive to healing. Consider the following example:

Negative suggestion: "You will NOT be able to put the tip of your tongue into the empty socket left by the extracted tooth."

Positive suggestion: "The tip of your tongue will feel drawn to the inner surface of your lower front teeth, just as if there were two magnets working to attract each other. When contact is made, you may experience a pleasant taste from the saliva released from your mouth. Let the contact remain until the tension is released and then your tongue will be able to rest for a long time before the tension recurs. In the meantime, the released saliva will increase the healing action in your lower jaw."

Notice that the negative suggestion does not define a desired action. Instead, it focuses on the problem and on controlling it with sheer will. The positive formulation, on the other hand, describes clearly what to do and provides therapeutic imagery in support of that action without involving an active struggle.

Minimizing Use of "Try"

"Try" implies uncertainty about an action, either about the capacity to carry it out or about the outcome. It should therefore be avoided when the therapist wishes to convey the idea of a successful experience. "Try" may be used, however, when the therapist wishes to imply that an action is impossible, as in the following eye-closing example: "When you feel that your eyelids are locked tight, try to open them. Experience how hard it is to get them open. The harder you try, the more tightly they want to seal themselves shut."

Integrating Suggestions with Ongoing Behavioral Cues

The credibility and acceptability of a suggestion is enhanced if it can be related to an event that is already occurring. Instead of demanding a particular behavior, the therapist capitalizes on what the client gives evidence of being able and willing to do. The following example of eyelids closing will help to clarify this guideline[1]:

"In a little while, you may become aware of your eyelids beginning to feel heavy . . . As they begin to feel heavy, let them close just a little bit . . . That's good. You notice how your eyelids have closed a

---

1. In this example, and throughout the book, ellipses indicate that the therapist's suggestions are made with appropriate pauses and cadences.

bit and that they are now beginning to feel heavier and heavier . . . The muscles seem to want to relax even further. How quiet and relaxed you feel as your eyelids close. The eyelids will want to close more and more as they grow heavier and heavier. Now they are feeling so heavy and they are almost closed. In just a few moments, they will close completely and you will feel yourself drifting into a quiet state. . . ."

Linking Desired Action with Positive Affect

The effectiveness of a suggestion is enhanced if it is associated with a positive experience. This general principle is illustrated in the previous example. The linkage can be emphasized, as in the following:

"As your eyelids begin to close, let this relaxation of the eyelids be accompanied by a feeling of warmth and relaxation in your shoulders and arms, with tension in your face and jaws decreasing. . . ."

Employing Indirect as Well as Direct Suggestions

An indirect suggestion is helpful when the therapist wishes to avoid having the client confront uncertainties about his or her ability to manage. As an example, consider the two alternatives in the case of a patient's need for reassurance just prior to surgery:

Direct suggestion: "You will be fine. I will be there, as will the rest of the team. This surgery has been done very successfully with many patients in this hospital," etc.

Indirect suggestion: "You know, a great many patients wake up quite hungry from the surgery and ask for unusual things to eat. Most of the time there is no reason why they can't have their preferences, but sometimes we have to offer an alternative because of the body's needs. Do you have some unusual food preference? The new techniques of anesthesia are so good that it is remarkable what patients want to do just as soon as they are fully awake," etc.

Both of these are reassuring therapeutic suggestions, but the indirect suggestion places the focus upon a very different issue, as if it were the central concern, and addresses the patient's unspoken doubts and fears indirectly.

Identifying "Markers" for the Experience of Trance

In learning about the experience of hypnosis, it is helpful for the client to become aware when he or she is in trance. In the following example, the induction makes use of the readiness of the client to keep his or her eyes tightly shut:

"That's good. When your eyelids close, let them feel as if they were continuing this closing process until they are tightly shut . . . The tighter you feel your eyelids to be sealed shut, the more resistant they will feel toward being opened . . . When you feel that your eyelids are locked tight, try to open them. Experience how hard it is to get them open . . . The harder you try, the more tightly they want to seal themselves shut. Very good . . . Now let your eyes relax, let yourself relax . . . Let your eyelids feel as if they were resting and that they could be opened any time that you decided you wanted to open them."

The fact that the muscle tension required to keep one's eyes tightly shut makes it dufficult to readily open one's eyes helps the client to become more confident in his or her ability to experience hypnosis once the difficulty has been encountered. This fact can also be shared with the client.

Repeating Suggestions

The quiet repetition of an idea, in the same or a similar form, is often helpful in pacing the suggestion. It seems to heighten the effectiveness of the suggestion by giving the client the time and reinforcement needed to absorb it within his or her personal state and readiness to move forward.

Utilizing the Client's Experiences

Incorporating the client's past experiences into the hypnotherapeutic process increases the client's readiness to go into trance and to make therapeutic use of what transpires. For example, instead of projecting a fantasy of relaxation, the therapist can ask the client to describe a setting where he or she has experienced a profound sense of quiet and peacefulness. Then, when the client has described the scene, the therapist can offer suggestions to deepen the relaxation based upon what the client has shared. For example:

"As the tightness in your shoulders begins to loosen, let your thoughts take you to the back porch you described extending over the water, and begin to hear the water lapping against the wooden supports."

Utilizing the client's experiences, and being guided by the client in general, come more easily to the therapist who regards the client as having the inner resources for knowing and learning how best to change, albeit with the aid (but *only* with the aid) of the therapist.

Formulating Suggestions Permissively

When the therapist's values and theory of change are oriented toward client comanagement of therapy, then there is continuous support for increased client self-management at every stage of the treatment process. Permissiveness, rather than coerciveness of suggestions, becomes a characteristic part of the therapy. A request for permission from the client for a change to occur may be implicit or explicit in the way the particular suggestion is expressed. Additionally, the client is encouraged explicitly to accept or reject the suggestion.

The permissive context of the suggestion generally minimizes that sense of coercion and feared domination by the therapist that many clients easily develop in the unequal power-field situation characteristic of therapy. It does not matter that this power relationship may have been sought out by the client for the purpose of therapy; it neverthelesss is feared because of a sense of the self's weakness. The permissive mode of proceeding is also compatible with cultural values that encourage rebellion when behavior guidance is seen as behavior coercion.

However, not all suggestions can be couched permissively for all individuals in all situations and still have therapeutic effectiveness. There are times when the power of the suggestion for therapeutic effectiveness may depend upon authoritative dominance. But these are, by far, less frequent. Much more typically, the permissive framework contributes significantly to the effectiveness of the therapeutic suggestion. It makes use of the client's readiness to accept responsibility for change.

IDEOMOTOR FINGER SIGNALING AND SIGNALING WITH THE CHEVREUL PENDULUM: EXAMPLES OF PROCEDURES

It is desirable to establish a procedure that will provide the client with a means of communicating attitudes that are less conscious or are ambivalent toward hypnosis or toward exploring particular problems in therapy. Ideomotor methods of signaling are admirably suited for this purpose. They are based on the fact that thoughts, ideas, and feelings are accompanied by involuntary muscle movements that can be amplified and perceived under certain conditions. Two ideomotor methods are described below: finger signaling, and signaling with the use of the Chevreul pendulum. In both cases, the therapist first introduces the notion of the "inner or nonconscious part of the mind."

In the following protocol, the therapist explains the purpose of tapping the inner part of the mind as a means of verifying the client's willingness to explore particular areas of concern. In this way, the comanaging role relationship of client and therapist is reinforced. Notice how carefully the therapist shares information with the client about the nature and reality of ideomotor communication:

"I am going to ask a part of yourself that is not identical with your usual aware mind whether it would be acceptable for you to explore [the therapist inserts the client's problem or concern] at this time. I know that you have expressed an interest in working on this problem because you made the conscious decision to seek help. However, you probably know that there are many things that we do, and even ways that we feel, that go on without our being directly aware of them. For example, you can sign your name without ever having to think of any of the small motions that make it possible. There is a part of our mind that keeps on 'knowing' even when we are not doing something with the conscious part of our mind. This part of our mind is referred to as the 'inner part of our mind,' where much knowledge that we have about ourselves is stored.

"Now sometimes the inner part of our mind may have judgments and opinions that are not identical with the judgments and decisions that the 'up-front,' conscious part of our mind may be experiencing. At other times there may be agreement. It may be most helpful, at times, to know how this inner part of our mind judges a given situation. One way that seems to tap the inner part of our mind is to let the managing part of our mind that controls our voluntary finger movements to relinquish control over the fingers temporarily, and to give control to the inner part of the mind. It seems as though the inner part of our mind, encouraged by this relinquishment, can express itself meaningfully through nonvolitional movement of the fingers."

Where *finger signaling* is the method of choice, the therapist can proceed as in the following protocol. Notice how the therapist assists the client in establishing the four finger movements:

"I am going to ask the inner part of your mind to please respond to what I will be asking by the use of finger signals. If the response is 'yes,' your right index finger will move up as if it were being lifted by a string attached to it. I am going to touch your right index finger and move it up as if a string were attached to it from the outside so that you will experience how it feels. [The therapist gently raises the right-hand index finger to demonstrate the "as-if" experience of the finger being lifted by an external force. This emphasizes the "nonvolitional" aspect of the act. Since the finger is actually lifted by the therapist, the client is not required to exercise any act of volition in order for the movement to occur.]

"If the inner part of your mind wishes to express a 'no,' or negative opinion or judgment, the index finger of your left hand will feel as if a string were attached to it, lifting it up. I am going to lift the index finger of your left hand in order for you to experience how this would feel.

"The inner part of your mind can also express uncertainty or insufficient knowledge by raising the thumb of the right hand. I will lift the thumb of the right hand, and the inner part of your mind can use this to indicate 'I do not know.'

"Finally, the inner part of your mind must be free at all times, without any need of explanation, to express the opinion, 'I do not choose to answer.' For reasons important to yourself and to your continued well-being, this response may be the most appropriate in response to a given question at a given moment in your life experience. When the inner part of your mind chooses to answer in that way, the thumb of your left hand will rise as if a string were attached to it, moving it from the outside."

The therapist then repeats the question about the use of hypnosis to explore the given problem and awaits the finger signal for guidance from the client.

The second method of ideomotor signaling involves the *Chevreul pendulum*. This is a round ball suspended from a chain. When the chain is held lightly between the thumb and index finger, the motion of the pendulum amplifies the small muscle movements of the fingers.

The therapist introduces the idea of the inner part of the mind as previously described. The client, with elbow resting comfortably on the arm of the chair, is then asked to hold the chain of the pendulum lightly between the two fingers. Four separate movements of the pendulum are shown to the client: Two of them are at right angles to each other in the horizontal plane, and the other two are movements clockwise and counterclockwise. Just as in the case of finger signaling, each of the movements represents a different response: namely, "yes," "no," "I don't know," and "I don't choose to answer." The coordination of a particular response to a particular movement can be left up to the client simply by asking the client to think of each response in turn and to allow the pendulum to assume a corresponding direction. Sometimes the therapist can help to establish a clear connection between a particular response and movement of the pendulum by manually moving the pendulum in one of the directions as the client thinks the indicated response. Following the establishment of the four movements, the therapist asks the client to allow the inner part of the client's mind to move the pendulum in response to a question posed by the therapist. An example of how the Chevreul pendulum was used in one case is given on pages 209–210.

Both of these ideomotor methods can be considered when a nonvolitional and nonverbal mode of responding is desired. The startling way in which the Chevreul pendulum reacts to thought responses can serve to convince the client of the potential usefulness of the hypnotic experience in general. The pendulum is typically used in the waking state, although it can also be used in states of quiet relaxation and light trance. Finger signaling, on the other hand, can be used throughout a wider range of states, even during deep trance.

The following chapter introduces the reader to a variety of approaches to help the client become adept at experiencing different levels of trance consciousness.

Trance Induction and Enhancement

The trance-induction experience provides the client with a shift of consciousness from the normal waking state toward a state where physical tension is reduced, where the individual is encourraged to be less critical of the self and the immediate environment, where attention has been turned inward, and where there has been a substantial decrease in outside stimulation.

Some writers have separated trance-induction procedures from procedures that have been called "trance deepening" or "trance enhancement." The following presentation does not make this separation since the deepening process is so intimately a part of the induction process itself. The various procedures used give the client familiarity with different possibilities of functioning within the trance state, and with the capacity to maintain the state of hypnotic consciousness even though engaged in a variety of experiences. Usually, the process of trance induction and enhancement is not specifically directed toward a particular therapeutic goal, although the accompanying relaxation is generally helpful in that regard. The more specific therapeutic use of hypnosis proceeds once the trance state has been achieved.

THERAPISTS' STYLES OF TRANCE INDUCTION

Therapists vary widely in the manner in which they induce trance, regardless of the particular method chosen. Some therapists prefer a stance of power and authority. They expect fairly quick compliance during the induction process. Pressure is sustained by firm and definite instructions to the client.

Other therapists are much more inclined to use soft tones, slow speech, and almost lullaby-like cadences. They may pace their suggestions according to the client's inspiration–expiration rhythm. There are quiet intervals. The expectation is for a longer time for trance induction.

Some therapists place a strong emphasis upon feedback from the client, especially concerning whether the client is accepting the ideas and instructions in the induction process. There is then more active use of client-selected fantasies and motor actions.

It will become apparent that my personal style predominantly fits with that of slower pacing and client guidance of suggestions. To be sure, a therapist's style is molded to some extent to fit a client's personality. Some clients respond more readily to an approach that is highly directive, whereas others are able to participate actively in selecting and guiding the ongoing events. In any case, it behooves therapists to become sensitive to clients' responsibility and cognizant of different styles in hypnotherapy in order to discover those variations that work well for particular therapists in particular circumstances.

METHODS OF TRANCE INDUCTION AND ENHANCEMENT

The methods of trance induction described below can be adapted to the special needs and circumstances of each client. The therapist would be advised to become well acquainted with a few prototypes so that he or she can flexibly shift from one approach to another if a client seems to be having some problem with the ongoing procedure.

Progressive Relaxation: Example of Procedure

In the preceding chapter, muscle relaxation was indicated as one of the conditions facilitating trance induction. People may think they know how to relax, but everyday stress with concomitant muscle tension actually prevents them from doing so. The method of progressive relaxation directly teaches the client how to engage the quiet restfulness of deep, muscle relaxation.

The following instructions can be extended or condensed according to the responsivity of the client. As always, the therapist watches for signs that the client is making use of the suggestions and paces the procedure accordingly:

THERAPIST: Make yourself comfortable in the chair. [I use an adjustable recliner with a foot rest that supports the legs along their entire length. If possible, the therapist should have the client lean back part of the way, with the foot rest in position.]

[The therapist orients the client as to what to expect.] I am going to help you focus in turn upon each part of your body. You will become aware of that part of your body by heightening the amount of muscle tension in it. That will help you become fully aware of any hidden tension that may be there. Then you will be helped to relax those muscles, and put that part of your body into a quiet restfulness until all of you becomes deeply relaxed and in a state of quiet rest, leaving your body and mind feeling free and secure.

Let's begin with your feet. Bring all your attention to bear on your feet, from the toes, the arches, to the soles and the heels. Become aware of your feet surrounded by the contact of your stockings . . . their texture against your skin on the top and bottom of your feet . . . Feel the reflected warmth of your feet inside your shoes . . . Nod your head slightly when you have become strongly aware of your feet. . . .

Now concentrate upon the muscles of your feet . . . Very slowly begin to tighten them so that the toes begin to curl under, the arches rise . . . and the tension increases in the area from your toes to your heels . . . Let these tensions peak. Very good! Now just as slowly, gently . . . Let the muscles relax until all the tightness is gone and let your feet once again fill your shoes . . . Feel the warmth of the surrounding shoes and the texture of the stockings. Take a deep breath . . . slowly release it . . . let go . . . Now quickly, intensely, bring both feet to the same peak of tightness as before. Hold it! Let go quickly and completely, let your feet relax totally so that every bit of residual tension drains away . . . Take another deep breath. Let it go . . . Let the awareness of your feet fade away and your feet go into a comfortable state of quietness, almost detached . . . So relaxed. . . .

Now focus upon the area from your ankles up to your knees . . . Feel the weight of your legs on the leg rest . . . the pressure of your calves against the inner surface of your clothing, against the top of the foot rest. Let your awareness of the texture increase so that your skin can almost "read" the weave of the cloth . . . Feel the cloth against your shin, resting against it. . . .

Slowly begin to tighten the muscles of your leg from your ankles to your knees . . . Other muscles in your body and your feet may also tighten on their own, but let your full focus of attention be upon the muscles of your leg . . . Bring these leg muscles to a peak of tension. Now hold it there for a moment. Slowly let the muscles relax . . .

letting go . . . releasing until all the muscles are once again relaxed
. . . free of tightness . . . You are aware of the texture of cloth against
your leg. Take a deep breath, very slowly. Hold it! Now slowly let it
go. . . .

Quickly, intensely, tighten your leg muscles to a high peak of
tension. Hold it there for a moment! Now let go, let go, completely,
totally. Let every bit of residual tenseness in these muscles fade away,
drain away into the chair . . . just letting go . . . Take a deep breath
. . . hold it, and as you let the breath out, let the focus of awareness
move away from the legs. Let them drift out of consciousness into a
comfortable quietness . . . feeling somewhat detached . . . along with
the feet. So relaxed . . . so released!

Now focus your awareness on the area from your knees to your
thighs . . . back to your buttocks . . . and to your lower back . . .
Sense your clothing against your knee . . . and over your upper thigh
. . . Feel the texture of your underclothes as they touch your pelvic
skin . . . Experience your weight as it presses down upon the seat of
the chair . . . Feel the warmth of the seat against your bottom . . . the
return pressure from the back of the chair against the lower part of
your back . . . Slowly and gently begin to make these muscles tense,
from your knees, your thighs . . . your lower back and the whole
pelvic area . . . Bring these muscles to a peak of tension . . . Now hold
it there for a moment! Good! Gently, let these muscles relax . . . let go
. . . Feel the thigh muscles let go . . . the pelvis settle back into the
chair . . . your back fitting against the chair . . . Let all the muscles go
loose . . . like a rag doll . . . Take a deep breath . . . Hold it . . . and as
you slowly let the air out . . . complete the muscle relaxation of your
thighs and pelvis. . . .

Quickly, intensely, tighten up all the muscles from the knees, the
thigh, the pelvic area, the lower back. Tight, tight, tight and tense.
Hold it for a moment! Let it all go, completely, totally. Let every
residual bit of muscle tension drain away into the chair . . . Take a
very deep breath . . . Hold it for a moment . . . As you let your breath
out . . . let the focus of awareness move away from this whole area.
Let your knees, thighs, pelvis, and lower back drift into a comfortable,
quiet feeling . . . a dreamy, detached feeling . . . so quiet and so
relaxed.

Now focus your awareness on your chest . . . your upper body
. . . your shoulders . . . your upper back . . . Become aware of the
steady beating of your heart . . . of your lungs taking in and releasing

air as you need it . . . Feel your back resting against the chair . . . Sense the space between your skin and the cloth of your underclothes . . . Take a deep breath, drawing the air in slowly . . . Pull in the muscles of your stomach . . . Expand your chest and raise it to its fullest . . . Tighten your shoulder muscles . . . until all the muscles of the upper chest are at top tension. Hold it! Experience the full expansion! Now slowly let the air out of your chest . . . Let your stomach muscles relax . . . Your chest drop down . . . Press out all the air in your chest that is possible . . . Then let go and feel yourself relax throughout your upper body. . . .

Now quickly and intensely bring your chest, stomach, back, and shoulders back to a peak of tension, expanding as far as you can. Hold it at this peak for a moment! Let it all go, completely. Empty out the air, release and relax . . . Let your chest become very quiet . . . your upper chest muscles all relaxing and the tenseness fading away . . . each bit of residual tension draining away . . . Let your awareness move away from your upper body, and let the quiet, comfortable, detached, dreamy feeling flow through your whole torso . . . as your focus of attention moves over to your neck . . . your jaw . . . your cheek muscles . . . your forehead . . . and your eye muscles. . . .

Slowly tighten the muscles of your neck . . . and your jaw muscles . . . so that your teeth begin to clench down. Let your eye muscles tighten . . . and all the muscles of your face and scalp tighten up until a peak of tension is reached. Your shoulders will become involved as you tighten up, but that is okay. Now let the muscles slowly relax . . . Let your jaw muscles unlock . . . your teeth unclench . . . your scalp and face smooth out . . . Your jaw may relax so much that it opens partially . . . Just let it relax fully. Take a deep breath and as you let it out slowly . . . continue to let go . . . completely. . . .

Now quickly, intensely, bring all the muscles of your neck, jaw, cheeks, scalp, eyes, shoulders into tension. Tight, tight. Now let it all go, fast. Release your eye muscles, jaw muscles . . . neck muscles . . . so relaxed. Take a deep breath and as you let it go . . . let the awareness of your head and neck area begin to fade away . . . your face and neck becoming comfortably quiet . . . letting the detached, dreamy feeling drift all over your head and neck. . . .

Now finally, focus your attention upon your fingers . . . your hands . . . your wrists . . . your forearms . . . and your upper arms . . . Feel your hand slowly forming a fist as the fingers close up tightly . . . As the fist forms . . . the entire arm stretches out . . . and stiffens into a tense and rigid arm . . . Let the muscles become more and more tense until they reach a peak of tension . . . Hold it! Very slowly release the tightness of the muscles . . . Let your fingers unroll . . . and your fist come apart . . . the muscles of your forearm and upper arm relax . . . and your arms drop lightly upon the chair . . . where all the tension drains off into the chair . . . Now quickly, intensely, bring your fist, your clenched fist, your rigid arm and forearm back to the former high level of tension. Hold it for a moment and then let go completely . . . Let all the muscles go relaxed . . . Let your fist become soft and unrolled . . . your whole body relaxing so fully . . . and so comfortably . . . as the quiet, detached, dreamy feeling . . . flows all through you . . . helping you feel so floating, free, and relaxed. . . .

With overall relaxation, the end of the induction of trance is reached; depending upon the response of the client, it marks the prelude to the next phase of the treatment plan—for example, alteration of pain perception, modification of stress reactions, teaching self-hypnosis, or working on some emotional difficulty.

Number Progression: Example of Procedure

All of us have been conditioned since early childhood to relate a succession of numbers to the experience of change: Sometimes it signifies a progression of either increasing or decreasing intensity; sometimes it represents a movement toward an anticipated event. These number sequences apply to size, time, value, and satisfaction. Numbers are used to mark growth, the accumulation of resources, and the countdown of a satellite launching into space. It is because of this rich psychological meaning associated with numbers that trance procedures make such frequent use of number progressions to signify entering into and deepening of the trance state.

The imagery used by the therapist to serve as a vehicle for the number progression (e.g., a calendar, flash cards) may vary substantially, as will the direction and the extent of the count. No systematic data are available that lend support to one direction of count, or to a particular fantasy or imagery, as being superior to another. Some therapists prefer number progression to proceed from a smaller to a larger number (e.g., from 1 to 20) to communicate the enlarging scope of the hypnotic trance. Then, in the process of "awakening," the count will descend from the larger number to the smaller one (i.e., from 20 to 1) to convey the shift to the waking state through a waning of the trance state of consciousness. Others, with equal logic, reverse this procedure and count from 20 to 1 to communicate the decreased intrusion of wakeful consciousness and the deepening progression to a new state of conscious experience. Either procedure has merit. It is strongly suggested, however, that a given therapist consistently maintain the direction most compatible with his or her conception of the change process. This tends to minimize confusion for the therapist and the client, as well as to lend greater persuasiveness to the suggestions, inasmuch as the therapist has used this procedure successfully in the past. The increased security and confidence of the therapist provides support for the client on the new journey.

The particular image or imagery invoked in utilizing number progression is also flexible, but a few guides are helpful—namely, the client's comfort with the imagery, and the therapist's familiarity with the imagery and preference for its use. The client's comfort with the imagery is important. The presentation of an image that is dissonant with the client's experience or evocative of additional tension is likely to interfere with the process of trance induction and enhancement, as well as with the rapport between client and therapist. The client may then spontaneously terminate the trance state. The most straightforward procedure is to check with the client about a particular image by asking him or her to nod the head in assent, or to shake the head in rejecting the image. Soliciting the client's approval or disapproval also expresses the therapist's regard for the client's judgment. Moreover, it involves the client in the decision-making process and demonstrates once again that the client is encouraged to participate wherever feasible in comanaging the therapeutic procedures.

The therapist's familiarity and preferences also matter, because the therapist not only uses language to stimulate an imaginary experience, but also communicates emotional attitudes about the image and the total situation through inflection, tone, and other qualities of voice.

It is worthwhile to note that the therapist's vocal delivery may influence the client's responsiveness. A quiet, clearly audible, sincere tone of voice, indicating confidence in the procedure being described, helps to provide the client with some of the support and trust that is needed at this stage of the learning experience. The therapist's rate of presentation should be sensitive to the feedback from the client—the signs of lowering tension and physical relaxation (e.g., breathing rate; pulse beat as observed on forehead or neck; arm and leg position; finger relaxation). If the feedback indicates continuing restlessness and tension, the time between counts may be lengthened, and the relaxation suggestions may be repeated and elaborated to communicate to the client that the therapist is carefully monitoring the responses and adjusting the experience to the client's needs from moment to moment. On the other hand, if the client's behavior indicates a rapid shift from the waking state to the trance state, the therapist permits the numbers to follow each other much more rapidly, with fewer intervening supportive and guiding suggestions. Also, the extent of the count may be reduced in future sessions (e.g., to a count of ten) should a shortened induction procedure be effective.

An example of a rapid number sequence is given on page 44; one that is much slower is described below. This example is offered as a useful number-progression procedure with a particular image—in this case, numbers appearing along a moving sidewalk. There are many other equally effective images that may be used, additional examples of which appear in later presentations in this book.

THERAPIST: Now take a very deep breath . . . Good . . . Hold it there for a few moments . . . Release the air slowly . . . Feel the muscle tension go out of your chest and abdomen as the air flows . . . so naturally out of your lungs. Your lungs are relaxing and clearing out the waste gases as your chest relaxes . . . Once more . . . take a very deep breath and let the air fill your lungs with oxygen. When your chest has reached its full capacity, hold the air there for a moment. Notice how full and expanded your chest is and how full you are inside. Now . . . release the air slowly . . . along with the waste products of your body . . . letting your chest relax . . . and also beginning to feel your body becoming more quiet and comfortable. . . .

[The therapist seeks confirmation of the suggested imagery:] Have you ever been on one of the moving sidewalks that transport people between large distances at airports and other transportation facilities? . . . [The client nods.] Good . . . I am going to ask your fingers whether the inner part of your mind would like to explore taking a special trip on such a long moving sidewalk . . . Your right index finger rose up to answer in the affirmative . . . Very good. . . .

[The therapist elaborates the imagery:] This sidewalk is most unusual because it has very comfortable chairs on it. Notice that the sidewalk is not moving at this point. Seat yourself in the chair and make yourself very comfortable. As you look ahead into the distance, notice the posts at the side of the moving sidewalk. On each post there is a placard with a large clear number. The first number you will see will be TWENTY, and then the numbers will be in sequence until you reach ONE at the end of the sidewalk . . . As you pass each number, let yourself feel every muscle become ever more relaxed . . . feeling yourself become more comfortable and more dreamy . . . As you are moved past these numbers, a quiet, peaceful calmness will enfold you . . . Let your thoughts dwell on times when you felt secure and good . . . By the time your chair reaches post number ONE, you may find yourself more relaxed, calm, comfortable, and peaceful than you have felt in a long . . . long . . . time. . . .

Notice the button on the arm of the chair . . . [The therapist invites the client's active participation:] When you push that button, the sidewalk will begin to move and you will move along on the chair . . . [The therapist invites feedback:] Nod your head when you see yourself pushing the start button . . . Fine. . . .

TWENTY comes into view almost at once . . . Settle yourself comfortably into your chair . . . Let yourself adjust to the position that is most relaxing . . . Breathe deeply and fully . . . letting each breath act as a soothing breeze . . . quieting you inside as it passes gently in and out of your chest . . . Sometimes the sidewalk may move you along a little more quickly or more slowly than my own count. From time to time you will find that there will be an adjustment, and the numbers and my count will become coordinated so that we are together by the time we reach number ONE . . . NINETEEN . . . [The therapist suggests further relaxation:] Become more aware of your shoulders and head . . . Let them relax and feel so much more comfortable . . . EIGHTEEN . . . letting go, drifting more and more into a dreamy state where thoughts come without effort . . . where there is such a light and free feeling . . . SEVENTEEN . . . [The therapist introduces additional imagery:] Sometimes about here there are posters, pictures, and interesting photographs on the posts along the moving sidewalk . . . Enjoy them as you see them pass . . . They all add to the total mood of peaceful quietness, calmness, gentle restfulness . . . SIXTEEN . . . FIFTEEN, a fourth of the way along your journey to deep and peaceful relaxation . . . breathing slowly and deeply . . . your eyes resting comfortably closed . . . your back and pelvic area feeling more and more relaxed . . . a dreamy feeling flowing around you. . . .

FOURTEEN . . . THIRTEEN . . . [The therapist encourages deepening of the trance state:] Moving along, going deeper with each breath you take . . . Feeling more and more peaceful . . . quiet . . . secure . . . enjoying the sensations and the thoughts moving through you . . . being able to hear everything I say with hardly any effort at all . . . TWELVE . . . drifting deeper . . . ELEVEN . . . TEN . . . well along on your journey to becoming profoundly relaxed, comfortable, peaceful . . . free from the pressures and tensions of your everyday life . . . learning that your body and your mind can relax and permit your energies to renew themselves . . . Enjoy the unique feeling of dreaminess yet awareness. . . .

NINE . . . So quiet, so relaxed . . . your body releasing its heaviness and tiredness . . . so quiet and peaceful . . . letting go . . . letting go . . . EIGHT . . . SEVEN . . . SIX . . . So restful, so refreshing . . . FIVE . . . just a short way more to go . . . feeling yourself so much more relaxed with each count . . . FOUR . . . Dreamy and quiet . . . feeling so light and free . . . as if your inner space is growing bigger and more open . . . THREE . . . TWO . . . Deeply relaxed . . . so deeply relaxed . . . the tension lines on face and forehead gone . . . ONE . . . The moving sidewalk stops by itself . . . You are profoundly relaxed . . . so good to have let go and to move into this comfortable and peaceful state. . . .

The trance procedure completed, the therapist and client are ready to proceed with the therapeutic tasks. But what if there is still evidence, after the number-progression sequence is over, that the client is experiencing considerable tension or restlessness? The therapist has several options at this point. For example:

1. THERAPIST: You have certainly moved a considerable distance toward releasing the tensions you were experiencing. Let me ask the inner part of your mind if you would like to continue this relaxation process even further . . . The finger said "yes" . . . Now see me move your chair onto the sidewalk just in front of the TEN . . . Now, when you are ready, push the starting button. . . .

2. THERAPIST: There still appears to be some residue of tension in

your back and shoulders. I shall count from ONE to TEN and the sidewalk will move backward to the TEN position . . . Then I will count down to the quiet stage even more slowly so that you will have time to release even more of the tension. . . .

3. THERAPIST: You can open your eyes now and we can do something else to release even more of the tension. [The therapist then selects a different method of trance induction and enhancement.]

Eye Fixation: Example of Procedure

There are many variations using eye fixation as a procedure, and it is helpful to have alternatives available when circumstances indicate that a shift in the approach being used is desirable. A particular procedure for eye-fixation induction that is effectively used with many clients is described here in detail. It provides a working model that can be learned; it also serves to illustrate the more general principles of induction.

First, a brief summary of eye-fixation induction is given. The client is asked to focus upon some defined point in space, such as a light, a whirling disc, or a finger, and is then encouraged to assume a fixed gaze. The resulting eye-muscle strain is responded to by the therapist. The therapist refers to the presence of heavy eyelids and eye tension, and states how comfortable it would be to relieve this stress. A suggestion of how this tension may be relieved is then given, and as the client follows through, the suggestion is extended to encompass general body and mind relaxation. The suggestion to lower the eyelids is related to increasing feelings of release from tension. Closing the eyelids is then suggested as a signal for a shift of consciousness, for a change toward inner calmness, detachment, dreaminess, quiet—a hypnotic state of consciousness.

The therapist carefully observes the client throughout the induction procedure, pacing his or her suggestions to coordinate with the client's state at a given moment, and then facilitating further involvement in the trance experience. The therapist's positive suggestions directly support what is happening, and also guide the client's anticipations and experiences. As the client's sense of the credibility and trustworthiness of the therapist increases, the shift into hypnotic consciousness becomes facilitated.

The following protocol is typical:

THERAPIST: Please raise your dominant hand and arm so that the elbow-to-arm line is roughly parallel to the ground . . . Good . . . Now turn your thumb up vertically so that the nail is facing your eyes, while the arm remains in its parallel position. You may feel a little bit of strain in your shoulder . . . Now slowly bring your thumbnail closer to your eyes, following a line right between the two eyes, until the single thumbnail image seems to split into two images. When that happens, stop moving the hand in and move it outward until one image is established again.

Focus all your attention on the thumbnail. Fix your gaze strongly on the fingernail . . . Good! . . . Gradually, you will become aware of strain in your eye muscle. Your eyelids may want to blink. Do your best not to blink. Keep your attention and your gaze fixed upon the thumbnail. . . .

Gradually you may become aware of your arm and your hand becoming heavier and heavier, wanting to begin moving down. As the feeling of heaviness develops in your arm and hand, you may also become aware of your eyelids beginning to feel heavier, beginning to feel how comfortable it might be if they were to close and rest . . . How quiet and relaxing it would be for the arm and hand to come to rest and the eyelids to close shut . . . Feel the stress in your shoulder and arm becoming more noticeable as the arm feels heavier. . . .

[The therapist introduces additional imagery:] Imagine some beautiful, very fine, clear thread connecting the eyelid hairs with the thumbnail . . . As the hand becomes heavier and the arm begins to drift down . . . the thumbnail moves down and the pull on the upper eyelids of the threads seem to feel stronger and stronger . . . Continue to focus upon the thumbnail . . . Your eyes have begun to water and the thumbnail becomes less clear, but you know it is out there and as the hand and arm grow heavier and heavier, your eye muscles are also experiencing increased heaviness. . . .

Let the feeling of heaviness in your eyelids grow stronger and stronger, but keep the eyelids open until you feel that you are unable to keep them open . . . Everything wants to relax, your hand and arm feel so heavy . . . They want just to move down into your lap and become relaxed, quiet, comfortable. . . .

Your eyelids are almost shut, they are almost closed . . . letting go . . . letting go . . . There may be such a light, dreamy feeling coming into you as the eyelids close shut, close shut, closed tightly together . . . closed tight, closed tightly together . . . All the tension in the arm and shoulder fades away as your arms and shoulder relax . . . The eye muscles relax . . . Take a deep breath and hold it. As you breathe out, the remaining tension goes out with the air . . . The eye muscles are so relaxed . . . The eyelids are sealed shut without any effort . . . The dreamy, quiet, calm feeling extends throughout you. . . .

Feel the chair press up against your body as your body relaxes more and more deeply into the chair . . . At the same time, the inner part becomes so light and free, floating as if it were supported on a magic carpet. The inner "you" feels so securely supported everywhere and so free to move about.

[Number progression is used to deepen the trance state:] Look around . . . You may see coming toward you a sequence of numbers from TWENTY to ONE . . . [Several possibilities are offered to encourage the client's active participation:] The numbers may be on balloons . . . or whatever. I will call these numbers off to you and as these numbers move by, you will feel yourself becoming ever more tranquil, peaceful, calm. With each number you may feel strengthened to explore new areas, to feel increased capacity for living. TWENTY . . . NINETEEN . . . EIGHTEEN . . . SEVENTEEN . . . SIXTEEN . . . FIFTEEN . . . so relaxed, so dreamy and detached . . . FOURTEEN . . . THIRTEEN . . . TWELVE . . . ELEVEN . . . TEN . . . becoming more and more dreamy and peaceful . . . NINE . . . EIGHT . . . SEVEN . . . SIX . . . FIVE . . . the essence of being alive just flowing through you, feeling so relaxed and good . . . FOUR . . . THREE . . . TWO . . . ONE . . . so free of tension and so relaxed. . . .

At this point, the requirements of the therapeutic plan guide the activities. The client may be helped to learn posthypnotic amnesia, or the process of phobic desensitization may be begun, or some dynamic exploration of dreams may be undertaken, depending upon the orientation of the therapist and the needs of the client.

Alternative procedures for eye-fixation include the following:

1. Fixation upon some point of the forehead or the vertex of the head. This requires various degrees of eye roll upward with concomitant eye-muscle strain.
2. Fixation upon an external light source, or a thumbtack upon the wall, or a rotating Archimedes spiral, or a flickering candle flame, or a Chevreul pendulum held between the thumb and forefinger.

3. Fixation on the therapist's hand with fingers extended as it moves up and down before the client, with instructions given to permit the eyelids to feel heavier with each downward pace of the hands, and to experience increasing effort and difficulty each time the eyelids open to follow the upward movement of the hand.

It is probable that the perceived sense of "involuntary" eyelid closure functions as a bridge that permits the individual to move from the state of ordinary alertness into the state of altered consciousness called hypnotic trance. It is compatible with clinical and experimental knowledge to interpret the seemingly "irresistible" need to close the eyes as part of the client's participation in a dynamic interaction with the therapist in which the client has accepted the role of being guided from without the self by the therapist.

Different clients vary in their readiness to entrust a certain amount of ego functioning and reality testing to the therapist. The degree to which this acceptance occurs tends to be linked to the security a client feels in the situation and to the measure of help the client may anticipate from hypnosis and from the relationship with the therapist. The experience of "nonvoluntary" or "nonintentional" motor functioning, such as eye closure, seems to signal to the client that being guided from outside of oneself in a therapeutic relationship is acceptable and worth the risk. There begins a feeling of freedom to enter other imagined situations for the safe exploration of potentially threatening phenomena. The hypnotic trance becomes the "ground," the internal environment that opens up alternatives not otherwise as readily accessible to the client.

Arm Levitation: Example of Procedure

The procedure for arm-levitation induction assumes the quality of "nonintentional" response—that is, of a response that occurs because of some thought or image that does not include a decision to raise the arm. Thus, it provides the client with impressive evidence that he or she has been able to experience hypnosis.

The arm-levitation procedure is as follows:

THERAPIST: Adjust yourself comfortably in the chair. Set your feet firmly on the floor so that they are fairly close to the base of the chair.

Bring your knees fairly close to each other. Fine! Now, extend your arms so that your hands are above your knees, almost at the kneecaps. Let your hands be cupped and the fingers droop down loosely until the fingertips barely make contact with the cloth over your knees. . . .

Concentrate your attention on the sensations flowing in from these fingertips. Feel the surface of the cloth so that you can tell if the texture is smooth or ribbed or rough. Let the fingers and the inner cup of your hands above your knees begin to feel the warmth radiating from your knees . . . The warm air above the knees is exerting a kind of lift upward to the cupped hands . . . Your arms and your hands remain elevated above your lap just high enough so that when you take a deep breath and hold it, there is the very natural rise of the fingertips and the hands up from the knees into the air . . . The fingertips lose contact with the surface and move up. . . .

Now take a deep breath . . . Hold it . . . Notice how your hands have moved up into the air . . . Even with the first breath there may be a feeling that one hand has a tendency to rise a little higher than the other into the air . . . Slowly release the air from your lungs and observe how the arms slowly drift down and the fingertips once more come into light contact with the top of your knees. One hand may return to a position a little higher than it was before you began your deep breathing . . . Focus your attention upon the fingertips, the sensations from them, and the feeling of warm air rising up and lifting the cupped hands. . . .

[The therapist gives permission and offers control to the client:] You may find that it helps your concentration to close your eyes and let all the energy of attention flow to your fingertips . . . Whenever you feel like closing your eyes to increase your awareness of these sensations, let your eyes close . . . Breathe in deeply, hold your breath . . . Be aware of the rising of your arms and your hands . . . and with each breath the upward rise may become much higher and the return down even less so that one hand no longer returns to contact with the knee . . . Breathe out . . . Slowly breathe in . . . You are now aware that one hand is definitely experiencing a much stronger feeling of lightness and retained elevation . . . Breathe out, and as you breathe out, the hand will have its lightness fade away and come to rest very comfortably on your lap, and then the hand will take on added lightness and begin to move steadily upward . . . upward. . . .

[The therapist assists the arm levitation with further imagery:] Imagine a large balloon, beautifully colored, filled with lighter-than-air-gas . . . tied to a soft but strong string that goes around your wrist

. . . I am going to touch your wrist to indicate where it might be attached . . . [The therapist touches the wrist of the elevated arm and gives a slight upward lift to the arm to heighten the suggestion of lifting.] . . . Feel this balloon adding to the lift of the hand . . . Let the balloon become as large as you want to make it to give the lifting pull to your arm and wrist more strength . . . Take a deep breath . . . Hold it. . . .

Let yourself remain deeply relaxed, yet able to open your eyes as you let your breath out . . . Look at your arm and hand floating so gracefully and effortlessly out in space . . . Enjoy the detached feeling of the arm floating there . . . Let your eyes close . . . and let the upward lift of the arm continue. . . .

Begin to feel the arm and hand drifting toward your body . . . as if there were a magnet on your hand and another magnet on your body pulling this hand in toward it with ever-increasing strength . . . You may be surprised to find that where you think this hand will make contact may not be where the inner part of your mind is guiding this hand. . . .

When the hand makes contact with your body, you will feel yourself becoming much more profoundly relaxed . . . You will feel yourself drifting deeper and deeper into a quiet, peaceful, detached calm . . . an enjoyable kind of dreamy state . . . The balloon will begin to grow smaller . . . and your hand and arm will slowly move downward into your lap . . . feeling quieter and freer of all tensions as the arm moves downward . . . Your hand is almost in contact . . . closer . . . closer . . . Now feel yourself relaxing so completely . . . the balloon growing smaller and beginning to fade away . . . letting go . . . becoming so detached and dreamy as the arm moves downward . . . quietness . . . calmness . . . feeling a strong, good life essence flowing through your body and mind as you relax more and more. . . .

Your hand is now in your lap . . . Feel your body pressing down into the chair and the chair supporting your body as the muscle tension leaves your body . . . Feel the inner self becoming freer and lighter . . . as if you move about freely while your body rests and renews its energy . . . Let this inner self feel so securely supported everywhere and so free to move about . . . You may see coming toward you a series of numbers. . . .

[The therapist then follows the same deepening process as with the eye-fixation trance-induction procedure:] TWENTY . . . NINETEEN . . . etc.

Guided Imagery with Examples

Guided imagery is part of all induction and enhancement procedures insofar as words are used to suggest an idea that is then utilized by the client in imaging the corresponding experience. The further elaboration of imagery can be used to advantage in inducing and enhancing the trance state of consciousness in those clients who have a good potential for imagination and who are ready to make use of it.

In addition to the fact that guided imagery provides a method for establishing the basic conditions that facilitate the learning of hypnosis (i.e., client–therapist rapport, limitation of sensory input, focused attention, muscle relaxation, and heightened self-awareness), it involves the client in the kinds of psychological experiences that are highly related to further therapeutic work. Transition from hypnotic induction into broader therapeutic activity is easier if the induction procedure itself involves the main characteristics of guided fantasy. The hypnotic state of consciousness, with its detachment, dreaminess, inward focus, expansion of inner personal space, and flexibility to explore suggestions, is experienced during the guided-imagery induction.

The client's readiness to use imagination may be observed while preparing the client for trance. For example, good use of imagination is indicated if, during the sway test (see Chapter 2, pp. 19–21), the fantasy of the blowing wind is so strong that the client shows a readiness to move back off balance if not supported by the therapist; or, in the case of the arm-weight experience (see Chapter 2, pp. 17–18), if the arm on which the bag with the bricks in it becomes so heavy that it is held up only with the greatest of effort by the client. As the client reveals strong imagination, and also a fair degree of security in the therapeutic situation, the intermediary relaxation training needed to permit freer imagination to manifest itself can be bypassed, and the client and therapist can proceed directly to the engagement of the imagination. If the client does not seem to be able to make use of the guided imagery, there is always the alternative shifting to other induction procedures.

The therapist may increase the effectiveness of the procedure for guided-imagery induction by first briefly inquiring about a setting where the client has experienced a strong feeling of security, well-being, peacefulness, and freedom to withdraw within the self without interruption. The therapist thus obtains basic details about the setting that can then be incorporated in the induction procedure. Once the basic setting has been constructed from the client's description, the client can fill in further details during the trance itself. Support for the therapist's credibility in suggesting security, peace, and detachment in this setting is likely since the involvement is based upon the client's own choice and description.

EXAMPLE OF PROCEDURE UTILIZING HOME SETTING

An example of the guided-imagery procedure, involving the security of being at home, follows. The details of the surrounding had been provided by this client prior to the induction of trance.

THERAPIST: Adjust yourself comfortably in the chair. Arrange your clothing, your feet, and your body in such a way that you will feel nothing binding you, or holding you in, or imposing a constraint upon your moving about. . . .

Take a very deep breath. Hold it for a few moments. Let it out slowly, and as you exhale, let your eyelids droop down, and let them close very gently . . . very quietly, very comfortably . . . Let your eye muscles let go, and the eyes seal themselves closed so that they can remain thus, deeply relaxed, without any effort on your part. Just letting go. . . .

Focus your attention on the index finger of your right hand. From time to time I shall be asking you to signal a response with that finger. You will raise the index finger as a response, but sometimes you may be surprised that the finger rises to answer a question all by itself, as though the inner part of your mind was raising it without any conscious decision on your part. Let happen what may. . . .

Let your imagination take you to your path on the way home . . . You are a block or two from your home . . . It is quite late in the afternoon . . . The air has such a pleasant feel about it . . . You are anticipating getting home and relaxing . . . You know that there will be no one home until much later. Just before you cross the roadway before the street on which your house is located, let me know with the raised-finger signal from your right index finger . . . [The therapist waits for the corresponding response.] Very good. . . .

Look both ways before you cross the street . . . Feel the extra effort as you walk up the hill to your house. When you reach the top, turn around the way you do so often to get the reward of the view for putting out the extra work for the uphill walk . . . The trees and the houses are turning to dark silhouettes as the light fades . . . When you

are ready to go into your home . . . signal with your right index finger
. . . Good . . . It is so pleasant. . . .

The house feels warm and welcoming . . . It is so pleasantly quiet
. . . You will have plenty of time to relax and let the tensions of the day
recede into the past . . . Hang up your street clothes and then walk to
your special room . . . Close the door and walk over to the window . . .
watching the lights coming on in the houses . . . feeling the very quiet,
peaceful mood flowing into you as it does so often when you stand by
the window and watch night flow over the city. . . .

Walk over to your chair and settle yourself into it comfortably,
putting the support under your feet. Take a deep breath, and feel your
eyes relaxing and gradually closing . . . Your whole body relaxes
totally into the chair, feeling so heavy, but with a light feeling coming
into your inner space . . . feeling so free, floating . . . so dreamy and
detached . . . yet full of life . . . as if you were floating on a magic
carpet . . . free to move anywhere and everywhere . . . You feel your
body resting and recharging its energies . . . while this inner self feels
so free, detached, better able to deal with life's problems . . . Soon
you will see some numbers moving by you while you float on this
carpet . . . They will look as if they were carved of wood, and they
will go from TWENTY back to ONE . . . As each number floats by . . .
feel ever more free and detached. . . . [See pp. 37–42 for further
description of this deepening process.]

EXAMPLE OF PROCEDURE UTILIZING SEASIDE SETTING

In the next example, guided imagery was used to enhance the trance
state that had been induced by the eye-fixation procedure. Earlier, the
client had described a peaceful seaside setting that was then used in the
imaging. Through the previously described finger-signaling procedure, the therapist had obtained approval from the client to the
question, "Is it acceptable for the inner part of your mind to go back
to that particular seaside setting that you found so restful, peaceful,
and comforting?" An affirmative response indicated that the client
was ready to proceed. Observe how the client was encouraged to
elaborate details of the peaceful setting while in trance:

THERAPIST: [The client is already in trance, and trance enhancement proceeds:] Drift back through time to the summer two years ago
until you find yourself at the seaside. Let your right index finger signal

when you are back at the seashore . . . Good . . . It is late afternoon and you are eager to get into the house and go out on the rear deck that extends over the water, supported by the big heavy timber pilings. When you see yourself in that situation so clearly that you can almost smell the water, let the right index finger raise up in signal . . . [The right index finger rose up strongly and remained extended.] Very good. [The therapist suggests dissociation:] Let one part of yourself, the inner part, settle down comfortably in the chair near the deck railing while another part of you, the aware, seeing, knowing-what-you-are-thinking-while-on-the-deck part, remains beside me right here in the present . . . In just a moment or two, I shall lightly touch the base of your throat . . . Let yourself swallow . . . This will free up your throat and voice so that you will be able to talk and yet remain comfortably relaxed, dreamy . . . and more and more de-tached from any sense of pressure or tension. As you talk about how you are feeling at the seashore, what you express will help you become more and more completely part of the seashore experience . . . of being peaceful, relaxed, comfortable, totally involved in that situation . . . Good . . . Look around you . . . What are you seeing and feeling?

CLIENT: [Voice is quite low; speaks slowly:] It is almost dusk . . . I'm sitting on the big wooden rocker on the rear deck . . . My feet are resting on the lower wooden railing . . . When I look down, I can see the water underneath the deck through the spaces between the deck planks. It's almost black now in this light, with specks of white on it that move back and forth as the tide moves the water. The sound of the water against the deck pilings is almost like a musical drumbeat . . . like someone hand-tapping with fingers on a drum head. No one else is with me on the deck. The top railing is grey . . . Almost all the paint is gone . . . Maybe next summer I'll sand it down and put another coat of paint and spray varnish on it . . . The salt air takes the paint down fast . . . I like the grey color and the feeling that it isn't all new and shiny . . . Just resting in balance with the climate . . . If I started on the railing there would be so many other things that would ask to be done . . . The grey is so much more restful. . . .

I wonder whose boat is out there . . . They can never make it back by dark . . . There's not enough wind to even fill out the sails . . . The air is so quiet. . . .

T: Let that quietness grow . . . Feel yourself become ever more dreamy and peaceful . . . letting go . . . What do you see?

C: That was a real picture-book sun as it went from yellow to deep orange and then almost reddish as it hit the clouds just at the horizon line . . . The colors have faded out of the sky and the water . . . The boat out there is only an outline now . . . looks like a toy boat . . . My feet have begun to feel tired resting on the rail, so I've moved the old nail keg with the cut-out tire tread on its top under my legs, and they feel so much more comfortable. I feel my eyes closing. When I close my eyes, I see the whole scene of the sun going down again . . . Sort of dreamy, drifting, not focusing on anything. . . .

T: Continue to see yourself with your eyes closed. Breathe in slowly and deeply . . . Let your breath out slowly . . . Feel yourself becoming even more deeply relaxed, quiet, and dreamy . . . Let this image slowly fade away but remain easily accessible to you whenever you want to become more deeply relaxed. . . .

This was the end of the trance-enhancement procedure with this client. The therapist and the client then went on with the therapeutic work planned for the session.

There are many other trance-induction procedures that have special applications, in addition to the five general approaches that have already been described. Three additional ones are briefly described below.

Sleep to Hypnotic Trance: Example of Procedure

Some therapists have found that the procedure of moving from sleep to a hypnotic trance has considerable value with children in conjunction with an ongoing daytime therapeutic program. The therapist (or the parent trained as a therapist surrogate to carry out the procedure at home) talks to the child during the transition between sleep and waking, strongly suggesting better ways of feeling and behaving. The transition period is similar to a trance state, and the suggestions can be viewed as posthypnotic suggestions. Usually the procedure is carried out regularly over a period of time. It is possible that much of the reported effectiveness of the method may be related to the warm, friendly, comforting presence of the significant adult at the time of waking and the changed attitudes in the parent working with the child, as well as to the suggestions given while the child is in the "hypnotic-trance" state of consciousness.

More specifically, the therapist (or therapist surrogate) comes to the child's room just a few minutes prior to the child's typical waking time, leans down, and places his or her mouth close to the child's ear so that the child can hear what is said while still asleep. The following suggestions were made to a child who had begun to feel increasingly apprehensive about going to school:

THERAPIST: You are still asleep. You are asleep, but in a little while you will feel yourself waking up but feeling very quiet . . . Now your eyes will stay shut tight. You will feel very good and still a little dreamy . . . Let your eyes remain shut tight . . . Feel real quiet and comfortable . . . Today is going to be a very good day for you . . . You are going to feel so good all day . . . When you get up, you will enjoy getting washed, dressed, having your breakfast, and going to school . . . So many interesting things are going to happen at school that you will hardly notice how quickly the time goes by . . . When you come home you will rememeber many of the nice things that happened at school and you will tell me about them . . . It will be such a good day . . . I am going to count now, from ONE to FIVE . . . when I reach FIVE, your eyes will be wide open and you'll be wide awake. ONE, TWO . . . your eyes are beginning to peek open . . . THREE . . . FOUR . . . your eyes are open . . . FIVE . . . Your eyes are wide open and you are wide awake. . . .

The parent used this particular pattern of suggestions during the early-morning waking time, and the therapist worked with the child during the day using desenitization procedures and psychodrama.

Startle Method: Example of Procedure

With the startle method, the client is seated on a bed or elevated table with legs extended in front on the supporting surface. A small pillow is placed behind the client at the approximate place the head will be when he or she is fully prone.

The therapist directs the client to close the eyes, and then informs the client that the therapist is going to move him or her down to the pillow. The therapist places one arm behind the client's back in a supportive fashion, and the other hand on the client's chest in a pushing fashion.

THERAPIST: [The therapist moves the client backward slowly:] You are going to become more and more relaxed as I move you backward . . . By the time your head reaches the pillow, you will find yourself profoundly relaxed and deeply asleep and yet be able to hear my voice very clearly. . . .

[Then, when the client's head is about 12 to 18 inches above the pillow, the therapist suddenly releases support and presses down firmly. The startled client falls onto the pillow while the therapist, in a firm, insistent voice, says:] SLEEP! SLEEP! Go deeply asleep, yet continue to hear my voice.

[After the client's head has touched the pillow, the therapist raises both of the client's arms. Typically, the arms remain elevated in a cataleptic position. The therapist continues:] Soon your arms will become very heavy, very heavy, and as they begin to move down, you will go even more profoundly into a deep, relaxed, sleep . . . Deeply asleep . . . Yet you will hear me and remain conscious though quite deeply relaxed . . . and your whole body is falling asleep while your mind remains awake. . . .

It is obvious that the tenor of this procedure is authoritative and forceful, in marked contrast to the other induction procedures, which are characteristically collaborative and paced to the client's tempo. The startle method would be ill suited as an induction procedure for most psychotherapeutic interactions, yet it may be quite appropriate in emergency situations, where a rapid induction of trance may be therapeutically significant for dealing with pain, wound trauma, or severe anxiety states.

Confusion Technique

The main idea behind the confusion technique is that if the client becomes sufficiently confused in trying to follow what the therapist is saying, the client will give up trying and will more readily accept straightforward suggestions directed toward hypnotic induction. The therapist speaks very rapidly, and directs the client's attention here and there by presenting contradictory and confusing ideas. Eventually a gibberish effect is created. This technique has been shown to be effective when used by experienced therapists.

SELF-INDUCTION OR AUTOHYPNOSIS: EXAMPLE OF PROCEDURE

The ability to self-induce the hypnotic state of consciousness has major advantages. First, it is reassuring to those clients who continue to have residual concerns or misconceptions about the hypnotic trance as a dominance–submission relationship. The experience of control over one's own trance induction and enhancement may be more impressive than the therapist's assurance that the hypnotic trance is "your own trance." Second, it can be used to deepen the trance state and to enhance security while working with the therapist. Finally, it provides the client with a helpful self-originating therapeutic activity at home for tension reduction or other therapeutic work.

After therapist-assisted trance induction has been completed, the therapist asks the client whether he or she would enjoy learning more about the process of autohypnosis. The client may be in trance at this point, or in the waking state. If the client affirms interest through nodding of the head or verbal response, the therapist might then ask the inner part of the client's mind to indicate via finger signaling whether such learning would be acceptable. This double affirmation reinforces the involvement of the client in the decision for continued participation in the hypnotherapeutic experience.

The general procedure used in teaching self-hypnosis is illustrated below:

THERAPIST: Your finger signaled that it would be appropriate for you to learn how to induce trance in yourself and to use relaxation procedures . . . Very good . . . First, you will relax in a comfortable chair as you are doing now. . . .

Take a deep breath and fill your chest with the air. Let it expand your chest fully so that you can feel the muscles stretch . . . Good . . . Now hold your breath for a moment . . . Now release the air slowly and let your chest and shoulder muscles relax . . . letting go . . . and as the air flows out naturally and freely . . . feel the tension release itself in your muscles and inside yourself . . . Very good . . . Let your attention focus on my voice so that my voice remains clear and understood as the rest of you drifts off more deeply into trance with each breath that you take . . . It may begin to feel that all of you is concentrated into just the listening part of yourself, while your body, your arms, your shoulders, your feet, and the rest of you are just drifting into a quiet calmness . . . feeling so peaceful, so light . . . so free of any tenseness. It is as if your whole self is released from pressure, permitting your natural energies to restore themselves and flow back into your body with new energy when you need it . . . Let yourself go deeper and deeper into this relaxed state . . . Very good. . . .

In a moment or two, I shall take your right hand and place it on your left shoulder. That is what you will do when you want to continue with autohypnosis. It will be a signal to the inner part of your mind to quickly review all your previous experiences with going into trance in a very short time. You wil find that your eyelids become heavy . . . Let that heaviness develop very rapidly and fully, so that your eyelids wish to remain closed. Then take a deep breath and permit yourself to relax more deeply than even now . . . perhaps becoming more deeply relaxed than ever before. . . .

When you have reached the level of relaxation that will feel appropriate for that moment, your right hand will slide from your left shoulder and come to rest gently on your lap. This will be your signal to yourself to maintain this restful state of quiet, comfortable peacefulness for the length of time you have set for yourself for restoring your sense of well-being and energy. You may be accustomed to your own inner clock that helps to arouse yourself from a long sleep period or from shorter five- to fifteen-minute periods. If so, then give yourself the signal to arouse yourself after the given time interval has elapsed. Otherwise, you may want to use an outside clock or other timing device to let you know when the prescribed time has gone by. Be sure that the alerting sound is one with which you are familiar.

[The therapist inserts a precaution:] Any sounds, noises, voices, bells that go on outside of you, unless they should alert your attention, will have no effect upon your relaxed, peaceful state until the signal you have set for yourself occurs. At any time that there is some important emergency sound to which you should attend, you will use it as an arousing signal, and quickly become alert and refreshed.

In just a few moments . . . I shall count from ONE to FIVE . . . Shortly after I begin the count, signal to yourself to become completely aroused, refreshed, and to feel alert. When I reach the count of FIVE, your own signaling will also be completed.

Is all this acceptable to you? . . . You are nodding "yes" . . . Let me ask the inner part of your mind to signal with the right index finger whether this would be okay for you . . . The right index finger came up . . . and that is also an affirmation. Fine . . . ONE . . . beginning to arouse yourself . . . TWO . . . The muscle tone that is most usual for you when you are feeling well starts to reappear all over your body . . . THREE . . . Take a deep breath and as you blow it out, let your eyelids become lighter and begin to flutter open . . . FOUR . . . Your eyes are open and your lips and face are smiling . . . FIVE . . . Wide awake and feeling good. . . .

Well, how do you feel?

CLIENT: Just wonderful . . . as if I had been deep asleep and resting . . . I was surprised that I could hear everything you said to me and . . . [The therapist has reached across the client, taken her right hand, and placed it on her left shoulder at the word "surprised." Almost immediately the client's eyes begin closing, even though a few more words are produced.]

T: Very good . . . Let the full past experience quickly flow through you . . . Your eyes are feeling so heavy, they close, you relax, relax . . . relax to that degree where you have a full feeling of quietness . . . peacefulness . . . and comfort that is appropriate for you at this moment. The inner part of your mind as well as your conscious mind will gain more confidence with each experience of self-hypnosis you have . . . You will be able to use this small "island of security" to help protect your energies and to limit your exhaustion of resources.

[The therapist inserts a precaution:] However, you will not use these procedures to bypass proper rest or sleep . . . You will find that you can make use of these autohypnosis relaxation intervals to prevent escalation of tension as well as to experience self-renewal.

[The therapist inserts another precaution:] From this moment onward, however, *no one*, including yourself and myself, will have any effect upon your actions if your right hand is placed upon your left shoulder *unless* you give specific permission for this to signal going into hypnosis. It is important to include yourself because there might come an occasion when you might have to scratch the left shoulder with your right hand . . . Your scratching would not be a signal for you to go into trance unless you explicitly have given yourself permission to go into trance. Good . . . Now, give yourself the signal to arouse yourself. . . .

[When the client becomes fully awake, practice with autohypnosis continues:] Now proceed on your own and give yourself your cue to go into a fully relaxed trance . . . [The client, entering the trance state, is offered further encouragement and guidance:] That's very good . . . It would be most valuable for you to practice this relaxation and self-hypnosis exercise at least three times a day for the next ten days in order to gain a solid competence in cueing your own self-hypnosis . . . Now give yourself the cue for arousing yourself into full alertness and well-being . . . wide awake . . . Good. . . .

The competence acquired through learning autohypnosis means that the client has a new method for interrupting the escalation of tension, a new competence in self-relaxation. This increased self-control contributes to the client's experience of hope and growth, and to the readiness of the client to explore additional coping strategies.

TIME ASPECTS

Induction Time

The amount of time it will take to teach the client how to enter the trance state of consciousness varies greatly, whether it be through autohypnosis or therapist-assisted hypnosis. Some clients have induced trance in themselves even before they present themselves to the therapist. The therapist then needs to recognize that these clients are in trance and may teach them additional cues for systematic self-induction and arousal before proceeding with the therapeutic activity. Some clients may have unexpressed fantasies about hypnosis, with attendant fear and inability to fixate attention or begin the process of detachment. The time for induction is in great part then devoted to helping the client establish security in the setting, rapport with the therapist, and a readiness to become involved with a new and potentially valuable experience. Thus, induction times from 20 minutes to an hour might occur before the client experiences a light to medium trance state. Induction time can be expected to decrease as the client gains security in the therapeutic situation.

Most induction periods are very brief after the early training period—that is, five minutes or so, often less. However, individuals may vary from time to time in their ease of entering hypnosis, depending upon particular interfering factors that may be operating, such as conflict, noise, drafty air, or physiological stress.

Assimilation Time

The hypnotized person is not a robot who automatically responds to a suggestion given by the therapist. Even in the deepest hypnotic state, the client is not unconscious. Whether during the induction phase or during subsequent therapeutic activity, the suggestion must be assimilated by the client. This means that the suggestion is first translated by the client into personal thoughts and feelings before being utilized in client-oriented action. The time required for the assimilation process may be short or long, depending upon the interplay of many factors.

The way in which suggestions are formulated can allow for assimilation as a process that takes time. For example, when the therapist says, "In a short while, let yourself begin to feel . . . " the therapist is taking assimilation time into account. Also, in recognizing that assimilation time varies, the therapist becomes especially sensitive to direct and indirect feedback from the client.

The value of relaxation and tension de-escalation procedures cannot be overemphasized, whether they are used specifically to induce and enhance trance or to facilitate more focused psychotherapeutic work. All demonstrations in the remainder of this volume involve relaxation as part of the hypnotherapeutic process.

Before hypnosis as a state of consciousness is used in therapy, it is assumed that (1) the client had learned to utilize hynotic trance; (2) sufficient security in the trance situation has occurred; (3) the client, through the use of finger signaling or other means of communication, has indicated the desirability and possibility of attempting to modify the distress by achieving greater control of the problematic situation; and (4) some kind of therapeutic plan has been developed.

The next five chapters present a panorama of hypnotherapeutic approaches. The illustrations involve actual clients with a variety of physical and emotional problems.

II

HYPNOTHERAPEUTIC APPROACHES

Guided Imagery

Guided imagery, in its broadest sense, is used in all induction and hypnotherapeutic procedures. Even in the teaching of progressive relaxation, the therapist employs various images in suggesting, first, the tightening of muscles, and then relaxation and quiet restfulness. As was seen in the preceding chapter, some procedures for inducing or enhancing the trance state of consciousness use more elaborate imagery. Especially to be noted are the examples based on the client's own descriptions of especially peaceful settings (see pp. 49–52).

The present chapter shows how guided imagery can be used *therapeutically*. The first four examples focus on ameliorating the stress of particular physical symptoms. The fifth example presents a tape recording that had been specifically prepared for the use of a client who experienced overwhelming anxiety in a variety of everyday situations.

ALTERING THE QUALITY OF DISCOMFORT: EXAMPLE OF LEG PAIN

The following illustration shows how guided imagery can be used to assuage discomfort by reinterpreting its nature. It is taken from a case where it was important for the intensity of pain to become tolerable so that healing could be facilitated. Trance induction had already taken place. The therapist continued:

THERAPIST: You have described this pain in your leg shin as being sharp and piercing, like a knife point sticking into the bone . . . A very distressing and uncomfortable experience . . . It would become more tolerable if this sudden, intense, sharp pain were replaced by a pain that did not come so unexpectedly, that gave you time to adjust yourself to it when it occurred, even if the new pain were not exactly comfortable. . . .

[The therapist begins to develop imaged conditions for modifying the pain:] Now visualize the left leg as being covered by thick layers of cotton . . . going around and around that part of the leg where the pain is most often experienced . . . See this cotton secured to your leg so that it won't slip off . . . The cotton is so thick and matted that nothing would be able to pierce through it, no matter how sharp it might be . . . [The therapist paces the process according to cues from the client:] Signal with your finger when you see this clearly . . . Good. . . .

[The therapist continues building pain-reducing imagery:] Now see a sharp knife thrusting at the cotton layers, but it absolutely cannot penetrate through the cotton protection . . . You may sense the pressure transmitted through the cotton . . . It may feel like a dull pain, but it is mostly pressure and you are much better able to stand the amount of discomfort . . . When you have reached the tolerance level for this dull pain, see the knife being withdrawn from the cotton batting . . . The pressure is relieved, and the dull pain drops immediately. . . .

[The therapist gives control to the client for pain reduction and healing:] Now that your body does not have to prepare for the shock of the sharp pain, you will be able to use that spared energy to speed up the healing process . . . When the pain recurs, you can gradually build up the thickness of the cotton wadding so that the pressure becomes more tolerable and the dull pain continues to decrease. In time, you may feel only a sensitive area on the skin as the healing underneath continues.

SUBSTITUTING A LESS CONSPICUOUS SYMPTOM: EXAMPLE OF EYE TWITCHING

Sometimes a problem can be eased if the client becomes able to shift the locus of the disturbance so that it becomes less socially conspicuous. The client in the following demonstration was a 35-year-old man who had had a marked spasm of the left eye for several years; during psychotherapy, this had been reduced to a twitching confined to the outer angle of the left eye and left cheek. Because the condition in this attenuated form had nonetheless persisted for three years in spite of continuing psychotherapy, it was decided to make use of guided imagery in teaching the client to transfer the twitching to a less conspicuous area of the body. Following trance induction and finger signaling, the therapist continued:

THERAPIST: Your finger signals indicated that it would be permissible for the twitching of your left eye and left cheek to change, but not to disappear entirely. That's very interesting. [The therapist seeks further permission:] Let us ask your fingers whether it would be permissible for this twitching to move down from your left eye and cheek . . . past your shoulder, arm, and hand . . . to the small finger on the left hand? . . . Your right index finger suggests that this would be acceptable until such time as the twitching everywhere disappears completely. . . .

A muscular twitch is the end action of a stimulus to a motor nerve from somewhere in the central nervous system. [The therapist uses an analogy to physiological mechanism in the following imagery:] See something like a telephone wire or a circuit wire running from your left eye and cheek into your spinal cord and then up to some switchboard in your brain . . . [The therapist solicits active participation from the client:] What color is this circuit line?

CLIENT: Orange.

T: Good . . . Now visualize another circuit line going away from the central switchboard . . . down the spinal column and out through your shoulder and arm and hand . . . and ending up connected to the muscles of your little finger on the left hand . . . What is the color of that line?

C: Bright green!

T: Fine . . . Now visualize the operator taking a special line coming from the inner part of your mind and plugging into the socket that connects with the orange circuit . . . Soon a bubble of light will appear and travel down that main line . . . onto the orange circuit line, and come out at the left eye and cheek as a twitch . . . Now have the central operator pull that connection out of the orange circuit and plug it into the green circuit. . . .

Now when that bubble of light comes down the special main line, it will go into the green circuit . . . down into the spinal column . . . to the shoulder . . . down the arm and the hand and into the little finger . . . Soon a twitch will follow . . . It may not be nearly as strong a twitch as before, but that will be okay. When the twitch comes, that little bubble of light in the green circuit will disappear . . . When you first get started, there may be an occasional leakage of light into the orange circuit because it has become so well used, but that will become less and less frequent . . . The green circuit may also drain away the energy of the bubble of light more quickly so that it doesn't make it to the little finger every time, but that's still okay. . . .

[The therapist suggests equanimity:] You will find a great tension relief to have your face free of this extra motor action . . . and will begin to feel even more comfortable in groups than you have felt in the past . . . Once more, let that bubble of light come down the main line from the inner part of your mind, move onto the green circuit, and finally express itself in the small finger movement . . . Very good. . . .

EVOKING HELPFUL PAST EXPERIENCES: EXAMPLE OF SKIN RASH

Biofeedback research and the autogenic therapists have demonstrated that many individuals can learn to modify their somatic experiences (e.g., temperature, blood pressure, gastric flow) through imagery, especially when imaging experiences that have been associated with such somatic phenomena. It is a common experience to salivate when remembering a delicious food or to have the salivary flow practically cease when recalling a dry, dusty afternoon in the desert. Similarly, rapid heart rate, warmth, and other body experiences may be evoked through the arousal of past memories. Even though the intermediary mechanisms that make these responses occur are not known, the body changes can be observed and recorded.

Hypnotherapeutic guided imagery also makes use of the individual's ability to increase control of body processes through the evocation of the memory of past experiences in which the desired body reactions took place.

The following example is that of a client who was beset with a recurring, highly irritating skin rash:

THERAPIST: When you had this skin rash three years ago, you used to get great relief from soaking in a lukewarm bath in which you had dispersed half a box of cornstarch. Of course, when you are able to get into the bath water, you can truly enjoy the good feeling on your skin. However, there are many times, such as at work, when you cannot get into a bath to reduce the distress of the rash. When you find that your tolerance for the distress is becoming shaky, close your office door and give yourself an intense irritation-relief treatment.

[The therapist draws upon the client's ability to enter trance:] Close your eyes and give yourself the cue to relax and become quite drowsy . . . Feel your body becoming lighter with each breath that you take . . . until you get the feeling of your body floating in your bathtub . . . and the water is at just the right temperature and you can see and feel the cornstarch dispersed throughout the water . . . When you have reached that point . . . signal with your right index finger . . . Very good. . . .

Feel the smooth, cool particles touch and coat your skin at every point where there is any irritation . . . and as the skin is coated by these particles, feel the coolness and the relief as the particles draw out the tenderness and irritation from each of the rash bumps. As the discomfort leaves, the skin energy is left to continue the healing . . . Feel the active healing as the new cells on the surface of the skin replace the injured, irritated cells . . . See, below the surface of the skin, how the blood is actively nourishing the healthy tissue growing on the skin . . . and the skin irritation subsides and becomes readily tolerable. . . .

[The therapist then offers a posthypnotic healing suggestion:] Let this cooling and healing continue even after you open your eyes, for as long as possible . . . Each time that you repeat the exercise, the postexercise effect of cooling and healing regrowth will continue a bit longer. Soon you will not need the exercise at all, because the healing will have been completed. Give yourself the signal for arousal, feeling refreshed and comfortable.

DIRECT THERAPEUTIC HEALING: EXAMPLE OF PEPTIC ULCER

Clients' knowledge of interior biological structure and function is generally more limited than their knowledge of external anatomy. The lack of knowledge tends to sustain shadowy and unclear images of the internal organs, thus adding to the sense of helplessness and loss of control when dysfunction or distress occurs. Guided imagery can replace these uncertain, often counterproductive images with images that are directly involved in the healing process. Although it is not known how these guided images mediate the body's recuperative energies, it is known that such imagery-induced mobilization frequently occurs.

The illustration below is from the case of a client who had a peptic ulcer.

THERAPIST: [To the client while in the waking state:] You have been doing very well in reducing your general tension through your hypnotic-trance relaxation exercises. But you are still having some of these pain episodes. I wonder what it must look like down there inside your stomach? What are your thoughts about what it must look like down there?

CLIENT: I have wondered about it myself. My internist told me that it is like having open sores on the inside of the stomach that are caused by the stomach juices digesting the stomach. He said that there is some kind of protecting seal missing.

T: [The therapist makes use of the client's terminology:] I wonder if there is some of that protecting seal stored somewhere down there that could do the healing trick, but perhaps is blocked off from getting to the right place with the right stuff.

[The therapist then encourages a comanagement role:] If you were to go down there and look things over, you might have some ideas on how to help your body get about its job of healing itself. You know, nature spent a million years preparing bodies to heal themselves against hurts. How do you feel about taking a trip down?

C: The only thing that would worry me would be whether it might not make things worse if I were to go down there and mess around. Also, I honestly don't see how this could possibly help.

T: Doesn't that question and your uncertainty sound familiar? Remember when you first began your autohypnotic relaxation exercises? You know, we can think of ourselves as having two kinds of reality that we live with: One is the reality of the physical structure, and the other reality is our feelings and beliefs about what our physical structure is. Both of these realities work on each other and affect our health. Sometimes our beliefs and feelings have a big effect on how we feel and act; at other times, the physical reality is the dominant influence. Sometimes the psychological image seems to be the most accessible route for change. In your case, you have certainly done all the physical things that have been prescribed. An explorer's trip would be to see whether there were useful possibilities involving the mind that could be encouraged.

C: You're right about the physical changes since I let myself learn how to relax and began using the procedure on a regular basis almost like medicine. So there is really nothing that I have to lose . . . except some trying. . . .

T: [The therapist is careful to seek confirmation of the client's readiness to proceed:] Let's do the usual check with the inner part of your mind . . . Would it be appropriate, at this time, for you to explore the interior of your stomach to search for healing remedies? . . . Your right index finger came up very quickly and strongly . . . Fine. . . .

[The therapist makes use of the client's autohypnosis skills:] Give yourself the signal to relax yourself into a very profound state of hypnosis . . . Since you are going to have to reduce yourself in size so that you can enter your mouth and then proceed down the esophagus to the stomach, it will be necessary for you to become so deeply and profoundly relaxed that there may even be a kind of loss of sensitivity in that area you will be walking in, so you will not find any irritation because of your exploring . . . Help yourself to go deep . . . very deep indeed . . . you may want to send your dreaming thoughts off to some marvelous vacation spot that you enjoyed sometime in the past, leaving behind your physical self to be checked out. . . .

You may need various equipment for your trip down below . . . See yourself with the right lighting gear, boots, perhaps an inflatable raft, and a big kit of medical and repair supplies . . . When you see yourself at the right size and with all your gear together and ready to begin your exploration, signal with the right index finger . . . Good . . . You are ready. Describe your journey as you proceed. . . .

C: There was just no problem getting across the tongue to the esophagus. I am surprised to find a kind of built-in stepladder with handholds and steps built right into the side of the esophagus. It feels like going down a very large chimney stack. There is a pale light all around, which is real convenient because I don't have to use the lights I brought along. The sides are clean and smooth. The handholds are warm and the walls feel warm and kind of throbbing. As I get to the bottom, the light is still good and I see something like a split manhole across the base. I just found the bottom, which opens the hatch door.

T: As you enter the stomach area, look around. . . .

C: The stomach seems so huge after the esophagus. It's like a cave with a dome. The walls slope down to the base. It seems to be subdivided into hundreds of sections with slanted separators that go from bottom to top. There is a funny-looking apparatus in each section. It is not made of metal, but sort of a flesh-like machine that keeps molding and changing a mass of its inside . . . Fascinating. . . .

T: Do you see any signal lights or other indications that describe if the particular units are working well, or what the particular function may be? I'm not sure where they would be located. It might be that these units could respond directly to questions.

C: Yes, I can see green lights, orange lights, yellow lights, and two red lights that keep blinking on and off.

T: Perhaps the red blinking lights are distress lights. Do you think it would be okay to check them out?

C: These two units are working, but they seem overloaded. The mass in the center has some very sharp and brittle angles. It seems to stop and start.

T: [The therapist invites the client's problem-solving effort:] Do you think that you might check your remedies kit to see if you have anything that might help?

C: I have this large tube filled with a white jelly, and it has a device like a grease gun that I can use to put it right into the center of the working mass. The machines are really shaking, but the mass seems to be getting softer, and the red light is staying off. Now the yellow light is beginning to come on. Funny, I felt really tensed up until the yellow light came on and now I have a really good feeling of relief. . . .

T: [Again, the therapist makes use of the client's therapeutic images:] Each time that you take your special medicines, close your eyes. See the medications go down the esophagus past the special hatch door, and flow directly to those machine units that have red lights blinking . . . If there is any left over, it could go to some of the other units . . . It might be useful to hook up all of the extra supply of the white jelly you have with you to the two red-light units so they could use it until they are really working well.

[The therapist then offers an additional therapeutic image and seeks confirmation:] Before you leave the stomach chamber to return topside, you might hook up a "sensor" apparatus that would pick up the red light whenever it shows . . . Have that circuit go right up to your inner mind . . . Whenever that special sensor notices red, you would become aware that something needed care before it became big. How about that?

C: That would be neat. I'll rig something up. You know, the whole inside looks so clean and efficient that I felt bad when those two units were spoiling a good performance record.

T: [The therapist reinforces the healthy-functioning aspects:] I think that it was really good that you found so much that was right with the machinery units down in the stomach . . . With your new early detector, you will be able to take corrective action early . . . You may want to link up an "insistor" on your warning system so that you attend to the distress warning.

    Now . . . come back up out of the stomach, and come to the exterior and let your full size return. Notice how profoundly relaxed your physical self is, totally comfortable throughout your explorations. As you fuse together with yourself, signal yourself to become fully aroused. Be sure to remind the inner part of your mind to be responsive to the early-warning system even if your conscious mind should forget . . . Good . . . Now fully arouse yourself, feeling right and well.

INDIVIDUALLY PREPARED TAPES: EXAMPLE OF PHOBIC ANXIETY

The following tape recording was prepared for a middle-aged woman who experienced debilitating anxiety at the thought of going to a doctor or dentist, a store or restaurant, and so forth. When the anticipated anxiety became too great, she was able to calm herself sufficiently to carry out these activities by listening to the tape. She routinely kept the tape in her purse so that it would be available to her as needed. If she was in a situation that required privacy, she used earphones. She had practiced trance induction and relaxation procedures with the therapist in the past, and had described a number of reassuring scenes. These are imbedded in the relaxation process on the tape:

THERAPIST: [The therapist's voice is recorded on tape.] While sitting in a chair, as comfortably as you can, you can let your eyelids close, blinking a few times . . . and then very gently let them close . . . As they close, let your whole body gradually begin to have a feeling of lightness . . . a feeling of lightness with the weight and heaviness going out of your shoulders and your chest, and then out of your abdomen . . . just letting go . . . letting your hands rest comfortably . . . feeling the air going in and out, from your abdomen, from your chest . . . Then feel the lightness in your hips, thighs, and legs . . . Just let go.

[The therapist introduces the idea of relaxing in a bath, a soothing experience for this client:] Let your thoughts take you to your bath where you are so very comfortable . . . just the right temperature . . . and relaxing very comfortably . . . with the same lightness of your body just floating and yet resting there . . . Very gently, quietly, letting go . . . Going deeper and more relaxed . . . [The therapist mentions a particular sensation that had been referred to by the client in the past:] Letting your stomach growl when it wants to . . . It has a right to make its own statement . . . Just feeling yourself getting lighter and freer . . . Very light and free. . . .

[The therapist introduces the idea of Wendy, the client's dog, a source of great pleasure and comfort:] And then, after a while, when you are out of the bath . . . feeling warm and relaxed . . . perhaps feeling Wendy near you, resting on your lap, or wherever she fits nicely . . . Just a sense of quiet peacefulness and letting go . . . Feeling secure . . . A sort of gentle peacefulness . . . Going deeper and deeper with each breath. . . .

As you practice, two or three times a day, wherever you are, just feeling this free, and quiet, and secure feeling each time . . . then when you're very relaxed and quiet, you can go somewhere you want to . . . or take a trip . . . You can do some of the things that you need to do . . . or want to do . . . and enjoy the sheer pleasure of moving your body. . . .

Whenever you choose, you can spend ten minutes or twenty minutes or even longer, just letting go . . . feeling your shoulders easing up . . . listening to your quiet breathing . . . sensing the lightness and freedom of your body . . . There is no rush . . . There is no pressure . . . Just letting go . . . gently and quietly . . . So good to let go and not have any pressures or any tensions . . . Feeling good and whole. . . .

And as you relax, the inner mind is focusing your energy toward healing and mobilizing your health forces . . . not only for the health of your eyes and teeth, but for whatever else is needed . . . to heal, to recover your energy, to restore your sense of well-being and joy of living . . . Very quiet, very relaxed as you listen to my voice . . . going a step further each time that you practice going into this quiet

space of your own . . . You can choose whatever images you want to
. . . Wendy when you want her with you . . . or she may romp off
when you want to be free . . . Very deeply relaxed, as long as you
need to be. . . .

When you are ready to come back to the here and now, give
yourself a signal . . . then very gently feel yourself coming back to the
here and now . . . the calmness and good feeling persisting even when
you are totally awake and going about your business.

Subsequent chapters present many examples of emotional and
physical distress in which guided imagery is used in conjunction with
other hypnotherapeutic procedures. Their great diversity with respect
to both problems and approaches reveals only part of the potential of
hypnotherapeutic application. It is important to keep in mind that
there is no single, best procedure in relieving a given problem. That is,
how a problem is approached depends on a host of factors, including
those that relate to the client, to the therapist, and to their respective
situations.

Projective Techniques

Some psychotherapists use projective techniques to bypass the individual's "censorship" mechanisms and psychodynamic blocks. Projective procedures can also be used to explore interpersonal relations, to sort out confused feelings, to desensitize the person to anxiety-provoking situations, and to discover new alternatives for action. The procedures described below can be adapted to different kinds of psychotherapeutic ideologies in fulfilling one or another of these purposes.

THE STAGE SETTING

The stage-setting procedure rests heavily on guided imagery to facilitate the ability of the client, while in hypnotic trance, to project a stage setting that will be productive for exploring relationships, feelings, and potential action. Because of its great flexibility, the procedure lends itself to the inclusion of a variety of methods associated with psychodrama and other projective approaches.

The attempt to describe a "typical" example of any psychotherapeutic procedure is always problematic since the client, the problem, and the therapist constitute unique entities that, when blended together, differentially guide the therapeutic process. With this in mind, a general plan is laid out below to indicate the potential of the stage-setting procedure and the variations that are possible.

Example of Introductory Procedure

The client is asked to proceed with the usual method of self-hypnosis he or she has already learned (or is helped to enter trance if this is necessary) until a reasonable level of tension release is reached. Then it is usually advisable to make use of the finger-signaling method to reveal the client's readiness to accept hypnosis in order to explore a particular problem at that moment in the therapeutic process, as well as to motivate the client to make use of the procedure as productively as possible.

THERAPIST: [The client is in trance; finger signaling has just been completed.] The inner part of your mind strongly affirmed your readiness to pursue the inquiry. [Of course, had this not been the case, other avenues would have been pursued.] Have you ever been in a theatre to see a play?

CLIENT: Yes.

T: Good. This will be a special occasion. You will be going to a theatre where the entire performance is created especially for you. See yourself at the entrance to the theatre. When this image is clearly in mind, let me know by raising your right index finger . . . Fine . . . Now enter the main lobby of the theatre, look around to renew your acquaintance with the theatre, and then proceed to the orchestra level of the theatre . . . [The therapist paces the process according to the client's cues:] Give yourself a moment to adjust to the somewhat lower level of illumination. There is no one in the theatre but yourself . . . yet it feels quite comfortable and very personally special . . . Walk down the aisle until you are reasonably close to the stage. Move into the row until you are almost in the center. [The therapist solicits a cue from the client:] Nod your head when you are comfortably seated and can see the entire width of the stage. I am going to gently touch your throat, and in a few moments it will be easy for you to talk and yet remain deeply relaxed in the situation. . . .

Now see me sitting quite near you. You will be able to speak with me without interrupting your concentration on the stage. Let the house lights begin to dim and the stage lights begin to come up brighter and brighter . . . Let me know just when it seems as though the curtains are ready to be raised. . . .

Until this point, there are usually few variations. The therapist may encourage descriptions of the theatre entrance, the lobby, and so forth, as part of intensifying the imagery and the client's involvement.

The purpose of the psychotherapeutic decision to make use of the stage-setting procedure guides the choices concerning imagery development. The goal may be to help the client explore certain moods or emotional reactions, or specific interpersonal relationships or settings. The different goals require different imagery development.

Imagery Elaboration with Examples

EXAMPLE OF MOOD EXPLORATION

If mood is being explored, the following procedure might prove helpful:

THERAPIST: Notice the rippling of the curtain, as if someone is coming from behind the curtain to the midline separation to make an announcement. See the spotlight focusing upon the speaker. Notice the smile [or, depending on what is appropriate, the frown, sad look, anxious expression, elated appearance, etc.] . . . The announcer says, "This is going to be a most interesting presentation. The curtains are about to be raised and you will see a scene at home [or at work, at school, etc.] Thank you for attending."

 The announcer leaves and the spotlight fades . . . The lights go out . . . The curtain raises . . . Slowly lights come up . . . Describe what you see on the stage . . . Are there people in the scene? . . . Who are they? . . . What is their relationship to each other? What is happening on stage? . . . etc.

 The client's responses provide the basis for how to continue the psychotherapeutic interaction in exploring moods and feelings.

EXAMPLE OF RELATIONSHIP EXPLORATION

The following stage setting illustrates a useful approach in exploring relationships related to the client's problems.

THERAPIST: The announcer says, "The man, his wife, and the wife's father are all sitting around the breakfast table . . . A conversation is in progress about their difficulties with each other . . . Thank you for coming to the play."

 The announcer leaves, the spotlight disappears, and the stage curtain rises. The scene is a kitchen and you can see the three people sitting around the table . . . Describe the scene and each of the people . . . What is happening? . . . How does the wife feel about her husband? . . . What kind of person does she see him to be? . . . etc.

Further Variations

The settings may vary from being completely unstructured (e.g., "The stage is completely empty. Soon stagehands appear with scenery and begin to assemble a scene. What is it beginning to look like? . . .") to being structured and detailed with respect to time, person, setting, mood, relationships, and even past history. The characters in the drama may be suggested by the client, the therapist, or both, according to the particular problem or area being considered.

Many techniques shown to be effective in psychodrama can also be effective when hypnosis is used—that is, in hypnodrama. For example, the outcome of a conflict situation on the imagined stage may not have been satisfactory or productive for the client. After the "curtain has been lowered," the therapist and client can examine the action, the relationships, and the outcome of the episode. Alternative resolutions may be explored. The therapist can then suggest that the client "replay" the scene while in trance with elements of the revised script included, to see whether the outcomes are more helpful. Similarly, the therapist can make use of a "stop-action" intervention at any point in the hypnodrama when review, examination, or interpretation of the events may have therapeutic value.

So long as the client is an observer of the stage setting, the stage action remains, in a sense, "action at a distance," even though it may deeply involve the client. When the therapeutic purposes are better served by engaging the client more directly in the hypnodrama, the therapist can ask the client if he or she would like to go up on stage, become part of the cast, and participate fully in what is taking place. The therapist may indicate that he or she will accompany the client onto the stage and be present as a voice audible only to the client while remaining invisible to the others. A whole range of projective procedures may become incorporated into the hypnodrama, such as movement through time, flashbacks, change of scene, an "alter ego" provided by the client or therapist, and so forth.

THE PHOTOGRAPH ALBUM

The photograph-album procedure is similar, in some respects, to that of the stage setting, inasmuch as it provides many opportunities for projection. It differs significantly, however, in that it explicitly and directly draws upon actual autobiographical events in the client's life.

Example of General Procedure

After the client has induced his or her own trance state (with help, if necessary), and the consent to proceed has been given, the therapist may say:

THERAPIST: Did your family have photograph albums in which pictures of family happenings were stored? . . . Good . . . How were the pictures arranged? . . . Were the new pictures added like pages in a book, going from front to back, or were they arranged haphazardly, or in some other way? [The client responds.] I see, added on to the back so that the time progression was that the most recent happenings were pictured on the last pages, and the further you went to the front, the earlier the time period . . . I understand . . . [Of course, if some other arrangement were indicated, the procedure would be modified accordingly.]

See yourself seated in a favorite, comfortable chair, and help yourself to become deeply relaxed and very much into your trance consciousness. You have a large album of family pictures in your lap. When you are able to clearly imagine this scene, lift up the index finger of your right hand . . . Fine . . . Now see yourself opening the album at the back and beginning to look at the photos. As you turn the pages, you are moving back in time to earlier periods. Examine the photos as you turn the pages. In a little while, you will become aware that you are approaching a period of special interest and you will come across one photo in particular that has very special meaning to you. When that happens, signal by raising the index finger of your right hand . . . Good. . . .

Look deeply into that picture and let its details become very clear . . . Take a very deep breath and feel yourself going even more deeply into trance . . . As you release air, have your throat feel opened up so that you can talk and yet remain very much in trance, and the picture may begin to enlarge so that the total photo is almost life-size. . . .

Describe what you see in the photograph . . . Where is the scene set? . . . What is the date? . . . What is taking place? . . . Tell me about each of the people in the photo. . . .

[The therapist encourages the comanagement role of the client; finger signaling is invited:] Let's ask the inner part of your mind if it would want to go even further into the picture . . . It signals "yes," so let the picture become three-dimensional, as if you were looking into it from a large picture window, and see the people begin to move, and gradually you can hear what is being said. Now open the picture window and step through the opening. The "you" that will step through that opening will be appropriate for the time setting, while the present "you" remains with me as observer on this side of the picture window. . . .

The particular incident represented by the photograph is then explored: the events leading up to the situation, the feelings, the relationships, and the action that develops.

A specific episode often suggests a history of preceding episodes important for defining the nature of the relationships presented, or the self-image projected, or some significant feelings experienced. Thus, after the specific photograph has been explored, the client may be encouraged to return to the family album and continue the journey backward in time until another photo directly related to the experience just explored is found. The overview about the developmental course of events and experiences may provide a basis for reorienting the client to the relationships and feelings involved, so that alternative meanings can begin to emerge.

Example of Relieving Distress through Restitution

Sometimes a particular incident recalled by a photograph arouses considerable regret or remorse, in which case the therapist might proceed as follows:

THERAPIST: Freeze the action back into the photograph right at this moment, and cross back to the present through the picture window to your comfortable chair, and feel yourself becoming very quiet and calm. From the perspective of who you are now at the present time, how do you feel about what was happening, what took place at the time of the photograph? [The therapist encourages acts of restitution:] Is there anything that you would say or do now, knowing what you know about what has happened in the interim and the increased understanding you have of yourself, that you wish you could have done or said? Would you want to cross back through the window and have the chance to say or do what your present awareness indicates? . . . Good . . . Take a deep breath . . . Let the window open and see the appropriate "you" going back through the window . . . [If the client were to reject the offer, the procedure would be changed accordingly.] Signal with your finger when you get back to the scene . . . Good . . . Now say what you would like to say . . . Describe what you would like to do. . . .

Example of Assuaging Grief

There are times when a client may return to a photograph that pictures someone who was dearly loved but who has since died. There may or may not have been ambivalent feelings about this beloved person. The revivified memory may stir up feelings of grief, and perhaps conflicts. After the procedure just described to provide opportunity for "restitution acts" has been carried out (if restitution were involved), the therapist can be supportive and helpful to the client in recognizing the grief reaction, as in the following instance:

THERAPIST: . . . The death of that beloved person does not mean that the person has disappeared. That person continues to live on in you as you continue to live and participate in life. You can revisit and share your love with that person whenever the need to do so becomes strong. You experienced how close and fulfilling that remembrance and reliving was . . . When your need arises, find yourself a quiet and familiar place, go deeply into trance and visit once again with your beloved one. . . .

THE HYPNOTIC DREAM: EXAMPLE OF THEME ELABORATION

Dreams are an important part of psychoanalytic psychotherapy. They are one means of providing access to the "unconscious." The potentials of dream procedures, however, extend beyond psychoanalytic methodology when the dream is viewed as a fantasy elaborated by the individual from the complex interaction of personal experiences and cultural symbols. Since every person dreams, although in some cases the dreams are quickly forgotten, the basic experience with dreams can be stimulated under hypnosis for the production of "hypnotic dreams."

It may be argued that the hypnotic dream is not equivalent to the sleep dream. This is both an empirical and a theoretical question that is far from being resolved. In general, clinical experience suggests that the hypnotic dream is much closer to dreams reported several hours or days after they have occurred, as contrasted with dreams reported immediately upon awakening. There is no doubt, however, about the clinical usefulness of the induced hypnotic dream.

In psychoanalytic psychotherapy, the client reports spontaneous dreams. The induced hypnotic dream is not limited to spontaneous dreams, because the client, within the special permissiveness of the trance state, is encouraged to elaborate the dream using the full range of projective fantasy.

The dream theme to be elaborated may involve a relationship, such as with a family member, lover, or associate; an emotional state, such as anxiety in general or in regard to a specific situation; or a behavioral pattern, such as aversion, attraction, or aggression. The hypnotherapy may focus upon experiencing a dream that provides the meaning for a particular symbol, image, or theme that has occurred to the client in the waking state, in sleep dreams, or during hypnosis. The search for meaning through the free medium of the hypnotic dream helps to decrease the sense of lack of control that often accompanies the involuntary recurrence of dreams. Any significant theme that the client and the therapist decide has not been productive during "awake" exploration may become the basis for hypnotic-dream exploration, with all the permissiveness for associational fluidity, nonrestrictive logic, lack of structure, and time–place–person transformations possible in dreams.

The procedure presented below is a general one. Within it, the context and manner in which the hypnotic dream is developed and utilized in the psychotherapeutic interaction will, of course, be determined by the theoretical orientation of the therapist.

THERAPIST: [The therapist helps the client engage in hypnotic dreaming:] Take a deep breath . . . Hold it with your chest fully expanded . . . Good . . . Now slowly let the air out and feel yourself becoming even more relaxed, with the tension in your chest and back decreasing as you let yourself drift into a very special, quiet kind of state . . . Let yourself feel as if the active awareness of your body is withdrawing from the outside toward an inner part of yourself where your dream consciousness exists . . . Feel your arms and legs coming to complete rest, as if they were drifting off to sleep as your active awareness detaches from them and moves inward, within yourself, to the dream-consciousness center . . . Your legs, arms, thighs, and other parts of your body feel more and more as if they were completely at rest as your active awareness gathers more and more into your dream-consciousness center . . . Your active awareness will center itself more and more in your dream-consciousness center, except for that part of you that maintains continuous connection with me . . . Let yourself feel that dream consciousness become more and more active as your body rests even more comfortably than it would in ordinary sleep. . . .

[The therapist helps the client focus on the theme:] In just a few moments, I will ask your dream consciousness to become engaged with [the particular theme that the client has accepted for elaboration], which the inner part of you has expressed an interest in exploring . . . Now, when you raise your right index finger, the dream consciousness will elaborate a dream . . . It will continue to elaborate while your finger remains raised . . . You will be able to describe what is happening with ease . . . and as you talk, your dream process will continue uninterruptedly . . . Should the dream process proceed more rapidly than your description . . . you will find that it can go into slow motion until you catch up with it . . . Let your voice and description remain connected with me while you are fully engaged in your dream process. . . .

Should the dream involvement lead to a suspension of the communication, the therapist encourages client verbalization. Interpretation of the experience and critical self-evaluation are deferred. When the client signals that the dream is coming to an end, either by providing a verbal comment or by lowering the right index finger, the therapist usually makes the following intervention:

THERAPIST: Your finger has indicated that your dream is about to end . . . that it has ended. Now take a deep breath, hold it, and as you let the air out slowly, feel yourself moving into a quiet state . . . [The therapist invites the client's choice regarding posthypnotic amnesia:]

The inner part of your awareness may or may not want this dream to be remembered in the nonhypnotic state at this moment. Let us check with the finger signals . . . The "yes" finger indicates that the inner part of you feels that the dream is free to be remembered in the nontrance state . . . Good . . . I am going to count from ONE to TEN . . . When I reach TEN . . . your active awareness will have flowed outward from your dream-consciousness center to your arms, your legs, and every part of your body . . . ONE . . . TWO . . . THREE . . . FOUR . . . FIVE . . . Feel the full active awareness flowing back into your body, which remains relaxed and comfortable . . . SIX . . . SEVEN . . . EIGHT . . . NINE . . . TEN . . . In a few moments, I shall ask you to give yourself the signal to awaken yourself, to feel refreshed, to remember all aspects of your dream . . . Now, give yourself your awakening cue. . . .

The suggestion that the client become immersed in the dream-consciousness center "except for that part of you that maintains continuous connection with me" is most helpful for many clients. The explicit support provides a "security blanket" and a freedom to elaborate themes with threatening aspects. It permits the therapist to provide reassurance and support without interfering with the dream production. This is an example of how the dual participant–observer roles of the client encourage the client to become immersed in a personal and complex experience while being able to report it as if from a distant objectivity. Clients frequently comment upon the positive aspect of this "control."

DESENSITIZATION: EXAMPLE OF RAPID AND REPETITIVE MEMORY EVOCATION

Distressing memories, whether stirred by one of the projective techniques or by some other precipitating event, may lose their emotional intensity and impact through a process of desensitization. Desensitization can be achieved by having the client repeatedly relive the painful memory while the therapist offers suggestions to dissipate the emotional hurt, as in the following example:

THERAPIST: This time you will go through this entire stressful experience again, but it will occur at a much more rapid pace. You will experience every detail of the situation again as I count from TWENTY to ZERO . . . [The therapist suggests reduction of hurt:] But as I reach the ZERO count you will also note a significant discharge of some of the emotional intensity tied up with the remembrance of this episode in your life . . . Let yourself begin the experience . . . TWENTY . . . NINETEEN . . . etc. . . . ELEVEN . . . You are well into the experience and it is beginning to come to an end . . . NINE etc. . . . TWO . . . The episode is ending . . . ONE . . . ZERO . . . The episode is over . . . Take a deep breath . . . [The therapist suggests emotional calmness to dissipate hurt:] Go more deeply into trance and have a quiet calmness flow through you as the pain, hurt, and stress of this episode dissipate and decrease . . . [The process is repeated:] Let us ask the inner part of your mind if it would be helpful to once more go through this experience at an even more rapid pace, with an even greater decrease in the stored tensions that remain in some form right up to the present . . . The "yes" finger signaled that it was okay . . . So, once more . . . etc.

Desensitization, abreaction, or whatever one chooses to call the release process is beneficial for many clients in the assimilation and detoxification of past painful experiences that, in terms of the current status of the individual, no longer need to arouse undue distress. With repetition and reliving under hypnotic trance, the "alien" quality dissipates, the episode begins to assume manageable proportions, and a better psychological perspective about the memory evolves.

Time Reorientation

SUBJECTIVE TIME AND WORLD TIME

Anticipation, pleasure, anxiety, or fear, to name but a few affective states, can substantially alter the experience of time. How slow is the passage of time while enduring pain, the sleeplessness of a night, or heightened fear; how rapid the passage during an enchanting evening!

There is general agreement that it is part of the human condition to be able to experience differences between "subjective time" and "world time." It is also generally known that marked changes occur in the individual's judgment about world time as the individual moves from childhood through adulthood to the older ages. Moreover, the experience of time is not limited just to awareness of the passage of time. The human being is capable of dividing the flow of time into past, present, and future time, and of further defining time both quantitatively and qualitatively. Time has markers associated with events, experiences, or other units of existence, as if they were set out on a personal historical trail.

In the hypnotic state of consciousness, there is an added dimension of the experience of time—one that can be characterized as a greater readiness for fluctuation and change in subjective time than in the waking state. Perhaps only in dream states or in states of toxicity does there exist as much or more of such flexibility. Important therapeutic possibilities for various systems of psychotherapy result from this flexibility in the experience of time during hypnosis.

An example of the therapeutic utilization of time phenomena has already been presented in the discussion of the photograph–album technique (see Chapter 5, pp. 77–80). In this procedure, the historical time organization of an individual's life is represented by the photograph album. By turning back the pages, the client travels through past time, with the photographs serving as the stimulus for revivifying a memory of some event, actual or fantasied, that might have relevance for the individual in dealing with current problems.

Varied therapeutic procedures that utilize the flexible experience of time under hypnosis are presented below. They are grouped according to whether the procedure involves age retrogression, future-time projection, or subjective-time distortion.

AGE RETROGRESSION:
THE "DON'T CRY" PROCEDURE WITH
EXAMPLE OF A CHILDHOOD HURT

The term "age retrogression" is used here instead of "age regression" in order to emphasize that the experience is better understood as memory activation that may or not be an accurate recall; it may be a confabulation, or a total fantasy of an experience in the individual's life from sometime in the past. The term carries no implications of a literal "return" to an actual experience that has somehow been preserved intact within the neuromuscular memory system. It would be very difficult experimentally to demonstrate the possibility of establishing such a complete functional isolation of any given experience that is inaccessible to interaction with all other experiences occurring before and after the particular event. It is more compatible with present-day evidence to postulate that interactions have occurred, and that the apparent "integrity" of a recollection is not proof that it reflects the past experience accurately. The therapeutic effort is to help the client recall an experience under hypnosis as vividly as possible so that its relevancy to the client's present functioning can be further explored.

The "don't cry" procedure takes advantage of the fact that almost every individual has had the experience of being hurt physically or emotionally, and then being comforted by someone. The procedure serves a variety of therapeutic purposes. First of all, the client engages in an act of self-affirmation while in trance by identifying someone who was comforting during a period of stress. The recollection is self-affirming, inasmuch as being comforted meant that the individual merited positive nurturant action from another. Second, the hypnotherapeutic procedure gives the client experience with dual levels of functioning during trance consciousness. That is, the individual can revivify a past experience and feel the self as being directly engaged in the past event while simultaneously maintaining awareness as observer and interpreter. Third, the procedure provides the therapist with the opportunity for being comforting to the client in a way that contributes to the growth of interpersonal rapport between the client and therapist. Finally, the procedure offers the client a training–learning experience in age retrogression during which events can be partially recalled and relived, and then seen anew in the light of more mature understanding.

It is assumed that the client has already had some preliminary experience with trance induction, as well as with trance enhancement. Furthermore, it is desirable for the client to have given both verbal consent and ideomotor consent (e.g., through finger signals; see pp. 29–31) to the procedure.

The following example is that of a 34-year-old man who was hurt during his mother's absence when he was seven years old:

THERAPIST: [To client who is already in trance:] I am going to place my arm on your shoulder and let it rest there through most, if not all, the experience. I shall most definitely let you know if I plan to remove it. Thus, my arm will serve as a constant and continuing contact between us, no matter how deeply involved you become in your experience . . . [The therapist facilitates two levels of the client's functioning:] There will always be a part of you that remains right here . . . aware of our relationship. . . .

Listen to my voice as I say the words . . . "Don't cry, don't cry" . . . I will be repeating them many times, and as I do . . . let yourself drift backward in time . . . backward in time to when you were hearing someone who was important to you saying the same words . . . "Don't cry, don't cry" . . . It will seem as if that other voice takes over these words . . . and you hear it from that other person . . . and then you will continue to understand my voice as it is and be able to interact with me as you wish in whatever manner you wish . . . When you are in the situation where the voice and the setting become clear to you . . . let the right index finger rise up to let me know . . . "Don't cry, don't cry" . . . "Don't cry." [The therapist's voice generally becomes quieter, slower, and comforting. It does not have a commanding tone. The word "don't" is usually spoken with a rising inflection, in an encouaging and sympathetic way.] Your right index finger has signaled that a setting is becoming clear . . . What is happening? . . .

CLIENT: My knee hurts . . . it's scraped and bloody . . . I'm crying and holding my knee . . . I seem to be lying down on the grass near the sidewalk . . . I feel bad. . . .

T: Who is saying "Don't cry, don't cry?"

C: It looks like my Aunt Mary . . . It's not my mother; it's my Aunt Mary . . . [silence]. . . .

T: What is Aunt Mary doing? Tell me about Aunt Mary. . . .

C: Aunt Mary picked me up and has me on her lap . . . She is sitting on the steps going up to our front porch . . . My knee still hurts . . . she has a wet cloth and is wiping my knee with the cloth . . . It hurts but I let her do it . . . She has these great big black glasses on and they look scary when she comes close to my face . . . She is wearing the apron she always puts on when she visits us . . . There are oranges, apples, and other fruit cutouts on the apron. . . .

T: Where is your mother?

C: Mama is gone away . . . I feel bad because Mama is not home . . . Aunt Mary is nice but she does not do things like Mama. . . .

T: How did you hurt yourself?

C: My bike fell over . . . I fell off . . . The front wheel of my old blue bike got caught and I tried to stop too fast . . . Sometimes the chain acts funny when I stop too fast . . . Mama doesn't like it when I ride in the street and the sidewalk is all broken up. . . .

T: When did Mama go away?

C: I don't know . . . She's been gone all day . . . I don't know . . . She left after Aunt Mary came. . . .

T: Can you ask Aunt Mary about Mama?

C: I can ask Aunt Mary . . . Aunt Mary says that Mama went to see Grandma, who is sick, and that she couldn't take Jennifer [the client's sister] with her . . . Jennifer is visiting at Alice's house . . . Aunt Mary says that she is taking care of me . . . I feel better when Aunt Mary tells me about Mama. . . .

T: It is good to have Aunt Mary there to help take care of you and talk to you when Mama is away . . . You like her special apron with the fruits sewed on . . . She likes to make you feel better when you get hurt . . . [The therapist facilitates two levels of functioning:] I am going to ask you to leave the little "you" for a moment getting to feel better all the time with Aunt Mary's help, and ask the grownup "you" that is here in the present but may have a special understanding now, at this moment, when he is in touch with the "you" at seven . . . Why were you crying so hard? . . . Why did this special hurt come back to you?

C: [The client assumes the adult perspective while in trance:] Now I know that Mother was away for several days. This was the first time that she had ever been gone for so long, and Father was also not home. I don't think that he had gone with Mother . . . In fact, I am sure that he was away because of his work . . . Aunt Mary came and took care of us overnight . . . She was my father's sister and lived in the same city . . . Her family was grown up.

T: As you look back, you can see that the young "you" is feeling so much better . . . You have visited back to a special time when you had hurt your knee and your Aunt Mary helped you feel better . . . but you also know that there was another hurt going on that you did not understand then . . . and that had something to do with Mother being away for so long . . . Now the crying is over, the ouside and the inside hurt feel better . . . Let yourself move up to the present in time . . . All parts of you fitting together whole . . . It was good to be able to visit with Aunt Mary . . . Take a deep breath and hold it . . . Now slowly let the air out . . . When you are ready, give yourself the signal to feel fully alert, remembering all the details of your experience. As you arouse yourself, I will remove my hand from your shoulder.

C: [In waking state] Hi! It was so clear . . . so close . . . I could smell the special perfume or scent that Aunt Mary always used. Did you know that?

T: No . . . you didn't mention that while it was happening. . . .

C: I know for sure that I fell off my bike and hurt myself . . . but I feel now more clearly that somehow I was being more careless than usual. As if I wanted something to happen . . . I really knew how to ride that old blue bike with its bigger front tire and rear tire and the handle bars that wiggled . . . I'd been riding it for more than two years . . . and really could manage it . . . The scene was so vivid . . . I could hear you ask me questions, but sometimes I was not sure what part of me was answering . . . Right now my head is just filled with all kinds of memories that I have not thought of for twenty or more years . . . The thing kept fluctuating . . . Sometimes I was back there so completely that I felt that if you removed your arm . . . I would become the seven-year-old completely . . . but at other times it felt like I was here watching a private screening of something very personal and interesting to me on a TV set or a small screen . . . but at all times it felt very personal. . . .

The age-retrogression experience of this man exemplifies a number of characteristic phenomena. During the course of his description, he showed the typical shift from past tense to present tense. Changes in his voice quality became increasingly noticeable when the revivification became more intense. Changes in vocabulary usage also occurred to fit the retrogressed experience; thus the shift from "Mother" to "Mama." The therapist encouraged the client to visualize significant details, such as the apple and orange figures on Aunt Mary's apron, as support for the revivification experience. Whether or not a particular visualized detail was part of the true historical event is of relatively minor importance. What matters is that the detail was a significant recall of something memorable in some setting, which for the moment was compatible with the recalled event.

This client had had many previous falls from his bicycle, and undoubtedly had hurt himself before and after the recalled event. The selection of the particular incident, stimulated by the voice saying "Don't cry, don't cry," was undoubtedly multidetermined. The reassurance for the physical hurt was only part of the event; the reassurance for the absence of his mother was also significant. The client's comments in the posthypnotic discussion strongly support this inference.

The hypnotherapeutic procedure in this case was guided by the following:

1. The therapist actively guided the client so that the episode remained relatively "contained"; that is, association expansion was not encouraged by the therapist's inquiry.
2. While the client remained in trance, his adult self was invited to help clarify the childhood hurt.
3. The client was supported in the search for positive, affirmative aspects of the reexperienced incident.

FUTURE-TIME PROJECTION

Changes involving the perception of self in future time is the focus of another hypnotherapeutic procedure that has clinical usefulness in many psychotherapeutic approaches. The procedure utilizes the flexibility of trance consciousness to enable the client to fantasy a future time when his or her life might be better.

Two considerations often enter the decision to make use of this particular hypnotherapeutic procedure: The first pertains to the principle of "affirmation of hope," and the second to the principle of "protected practice"—that is, the opportunity for safely exploring new ways of living.

Affirmation of Hope in Future Time: Example of an Improved Relationship

Support of the client's hope that the future will hold some positive outcomes with regard to his or her problems is an important part of the therapeutic encounter, for hope is a major component of the client's readiness to continue to risk alternative ways of coping with stress and to work toward change. During the course of a therapeutic experience, there are times when the client may experience significant depletion of the resource of hope. Stress from ongoing life events may increase, the pace of change may be moving too slowly, or the loss of clarity of values or goals may bear heavily on the client. In such down-spirited times, as well as at times of therapeutic impasse or uncertainty, the procedure of future-time projection may be of considerable value for both the client and the therapist.

The very act of projecting a time in the future where present problems have been alleviated or resolved becomes a statement of the persistence of hope and the willingness to renew that hope. It affirms belief in the self, in life, and even in the therapeutic encounter. When no such future time can be projected, then there is strong indication of depression and of marked limitation in the capacity to tolerate risks of any kind. Change is perceived as more threatening than the currently experienced anguish, deprivation, anxiety, or conflict.

The following case of a young married woman presents the basic methodology of the future-time projection procedure, and illustrates the strengthening of hope. This hypnotherapeutic procedure would, of course, take place only after there has been an ongoing psychotherapy relationship and the client has achieved some competency in the use of trance consciousness.

THERAPIST: Give yourself the signal to relax even more profoundly than before . . . Take a very deep breath and hold it . . . Now, as you release this breath . . . begin to feel as though you were free to drift ahead in time . . . To help that movement through time . . . imagine a

wall calendar . . . a thick pad of pages . . . each of which has a date
. . . the day, month, and year printed on it in bold, large type . . .
[The therapist paces the imagery according to the tempo of the
client:] When that image is clearly in mind . . . please signal with
your right index finger . . . Good . . . Now . . . as you move ahead in
time . . . have the pages just detach themselves from the calendar
without any effort . . . coming off as quickly or as slowly as the inner
part of your mind determines while you move into future time . . . In
a little while, you will be coming to a time that the inner part of your
mind will know is a time when many of the difficult problems with
which you have worked so hard in the past have become easier or have
been resolved . . . You are feeling so much better about your own life
. . . Your feelings of well-being occur so much more often and last
longer . . . I am going to count from FIVE to ONE . . . As I do this, the
process of movement into the future will come to that definite time,
and your finger will rise . . . At that point there will be a date on the
calendar . . . FIVE . . . FOUR . . . THREE . . . TWO . . . The pages have
stopped their fast pace and are barely dropping off . . . ONE . . . Your
finger has risen . . . What does the calendar read?

CLIENT: September 4, 1976 [three years into the future from the
actual date of the therapy session].

T: Good. Where are you? Describe your situation. . . .

C: I am in our new apartment . . . It is late in the afternoon but the
apartment is still light and cheerful . . . It's a new place . . . John and I
have been back together now for almost a year and we moved to the
city . . . From the living room window I can see the red brick tiles of
the plaza buildings . . . Most of the furniture in the apartment is from
our old apartment . . . but I have a new reading lamp by my special
chair . . . I have just come home from work, but John is not home yet
. . . I began teaching half-time at the community college this fall . . .
which was about all I could handle after so long away from teaching. . . .

T: [The therapist reinforces the positive outlook:] Your apartment
and your life seem so much brighter and more cheerful . . . You feel
the capacity to enjoy things again . . . Do you remember back when
you had those headaches and those desperate feelings three years ago?
. . . What has happened to them?

C: I still occasionally have a severe headache, but somehow it is more
manageable because there are good times in between . . . Two Cafer-

gots [tablets for migraine] really bring the bad ones under control
. . . and then they are over by the next day . . . The relaxation
exercises have helped a great deal . . . My downs are probably more
than some people have, but I know they are not for always . . .
Having John back is great. . . .

T: Your life seems to be significantly better . . . This is a much better
world for you and for John . . . You may remember that three years
ago the situation did not seem so promising . . . Those down feelings
hung on for such long periods . . . But there was a change, obviously
. . . [The therapist invites insight from the client:] Something happened to change the scene . . . Looking back . . . what made the
difference?

C: I think it was when I actually began hearing what you were
suggesting about John . . . You had kept saying that John had to accept
responsibility for his own decisions . . . that I would not be able to
protect him from his own decisions . . . I know that you had raised
that with me before, but I kept on feeling bad when I did not take care
of him when he made mistakes . . . There seemed to be no way I could
keep from feeling guilty about John's difficulties. . . .

T: Was it helpful when our sessions shifted from their emphasis upon
your own search for recognition to a focus upon your protection of
John?

C: Yes, that helped . . . but it was so hard for me . . . I felt that I was
abandoning John . . . that we would lose our connectedness . . . that
he would take off. . . .

T: From your recall, it seems that John must have taken off . . . That
you somehow came to terms with that, that he took off, and that he
also came back on a different basis . . . Something new between the
two of you. . . .

C: It had to be something new . . . the old way was more than I knew
how to handle . . . and maybe John couldn't handle it either. . . .

T: There seems to be so much to look forward to . . . Now take a deep
breath, hold it. Look around your new apartment, out the window,
and let your breath out slowly as you relax deeply in your special
chair . . . [The therapist seeks permission from the client:] Is it all
right with the inner part of your mind for you to remember all the
details of this trip into the future when you terminate your trance
consciousness and enter your alert, waking consciousness? . . . The
"yes" finger rose up . . . Look on that wall calendar again and just

imagine a movie film that has been reversed . . . See the pages jump back onto the calendar as the time clock moves back to the present . . . I shall count from ONE to FIVE . . . When I reach FIVE, you will be back in the present, but somehow it will be a slightly different present, and you will remember your trip . . . ONE . . . TWO . . . THREE . . . FOUR . . . almost back into the present . . . FIVE . . . back into the present . . . When you are ready, give yourself the signal to become alert and fully awake. . . .

Not only is it clear that this client felt hopeful that there could or would be a time when her life would be straightened out, but her review of the sequence of events leading to the improvement also pointed to particular areas of concern important in the therapeutic process.

Protected Practice in Future Time: Example of Coping with Anxiety

The principle of "protected practice" is another utilization of future-time reorientation. The underlying premise is that it is helpful to the individual to be able to practice a new mode of coping in a projected future-time situation, when all complicating contingencies can be safely examined and coping actions rehearsed. When the time for action in the more immediate reality becomes appropriate, then the vicarious rehearsals and the practice have helped to prepare and train the person for new ways of dealing with the situation.

The big barrier to the use of fantasy rehearsal in the present is frequently the conviction on the part of the client that the problem is insoluble, that efforts to seek alternatives will be futile, that even if alternatives are found the end result will only be further disappointment. It is in such situations that reorientation of the individual to a future-time setting provides the interesting clinical possibility for the client to bypass the early therapeutic stages of self-immobilizing attitudes, and to become involved instead in the later stages of coping exploration.

The client in the case selected to demonstrate the application of future-time projection for purposes of "protected practice" was a competent woman in her late 30s. Over a period of two years, she had withdrawn more and more from personal, business, and recreational activities of various kinds. She had begun to experience intense anxiety reactions in church, in restaurants, when riding in an automobile with someone else driving, and so forth. She began to find it more and more difficult to go into stores and shopping centers.

Over a period of time, the client came to recognize the intimate link between her feelings of anger at herself and resentment toward others because she had so much difficulty in saying "no" to invitations from those with whom she had warm relationships. She began to realize that the tension and "sick feeling" she experienced developed in situations in which she felt trapped into entering because she did not know how to refuse the invitation. This recognition helped to resolve the problem of saying "no" because the fear of becoming agitated and anxious in public was greater than her fears about declining the invitation.

Unfortunately, the cost of the solution—to decline invitations—had become much greater than the original problem. It was as if the anxiety reactions had taken on a life of their own and spread to a very broad range of public settings. Even though she had made excellent progress in psychotherapy, learning how to say "no" to family, friends, and associates without fear of rejection, she was unable to say "yes" because she could not conceive of herself as being able to cope with the possibility of becoming nauseated and anxious in public. This seemed to be a relevant situation for using the procedure of protected practice in future time:

THERAPIST: [To client in waking state:] Most of your difficulty seems to be focused around the point of deciding whether to say "yes" and take a risk, and then enduring the waiting period until the actual action. Your finger signals indicated that the inner part of your mind was interested in finding new ways of dealing with this situation, since you would regain more space in which you have choices.

Good . . . Take a deep breath and hold it . . . Let the air out of your lungs slowly and as your chest relaxes . . . let yourself relax deeply all over . . . Just let go. . . .

Imagine that you are looking at a special time clock whose hand marks off days and weeks rather than hours . . . When you see this time clock clearly, signal by nodding your head . . . Very good . . . Now let that hand begin moving, and as it marks off the days and weeks, move with the clock into future time . . . into time that is yet to be . . . I shall count from FIVE to ONE . . . When I reach ONE you will find yourself right in the middle of one of those typical situations where you can practice some new adjusting techniques . . . FIVE . . . FOUR . . . THREE . . . moving ahead in time . . . TWO . . . You have skipped all the preliminaries of decision, planning, waiting . . . All that is past . . . You are right in the middle of the situation . . . ONE. . . .

Raise your right index finger when the situation and the setting become clear . . . Things have been under way for some time and you have managed quite well thus far . . . Good . . . Your finger signals that you are there . . . You can remain deeply relaxed . . . [The therapist encourages two levels of functioning:] Part of you is very involved in what is going on in that future-time experience, and part of you remains calmly with me right here . . . Where are you?

CLIENT: It is early May, and the fund-raising drive is over . . . and this is the recognition dinner that the Lyric Opera Guild always holds . . . Jerry is sitting right next to me, and he seems so pleased that I am here . . . The cocktail bit is over . . . and we're in the main dining room . . . Dinner is about to be served I have that sick, sinking feeling in my stomach . . . If I get up I will fall flat on my face in front of everyone. . . .

T: [The therapist encourages the client to take control by suggesting options:] But that is what is so neat about your situation right now . . . You can move the time clock ahead so that the dinner is over and done with . . . or you can move it back into the cocktail hour . . . or you can stay with it to see what can be done . . . You have many choices . . . Which one do you want to choose?

C: If I could just get outside of the dining room for even a short time . . . then I'd stay with it. . . .

T: How about the ladies' rest room? After all . . . there was plenty of fluid intake during the cocktail hour . . . Seems like a reasonable basis for leaving the dining room . . . How about it?

C: Okay.

T: So get up . . . Feel strong . . . Tell Jerry where you're going . . . And where are you now?

C: I'm making it out of the dining room on my own power . . . I know just where the ladies' rest room is . . . because that is an old habit of mine from way back . . . I always locate it so I can have a safety retreat if I need it . . . Made it!

T: Now you have more options . . . You can use the privacy of the rest room to do some breathing exercises . . . to meditate . . . to use your trance consciousness to calm your insides . . . Which will you choose?

C: I have my rebreathing bag . . . I feel that I must have started overbreathing without getting my warning signal . . . That's better . . . That stomach feeling is almost all gone. . . .

T: You were not trapped . . . Even if you didn't leave the dining room you still had choices . . . but you see . . . as soon as you gave yourself a valid reason . . . you could leave with strength . . . There are always valid reasons to be found or invented . . . Are you ready to return to the dining hall?

C: Yup! . . . I'm almost at the dining hall, but it is really a struggle to get myself to go back in. . . .

T: [The therapist reassures the client:] Of course . . . that's so understandable . . . Just before, you were feeling calm and good inside . . . In the dining hall there is uncertainty . . . [The therapist invites the client to take control by thinking of management strategies:] What would make it much easier for you when you went back in?

C: Two things . . . If Jerry and I were sitting near a door . . . and if there was an open window that I could see out of . . . just a glimpse of the outside would be enough to really open up that whole space for me. . . .

T: [The therapist complies with the selected strategy by suggesting corresponding imagery:] That should be easy to arrange . . . Look around the banquet hall area . . . See that table over there near the French doors that open onto the garden outside the dining hall . . . There are two seats at the table there . . . Go over and find your name cards . . . Those doors also have an EXIT sign over them . . . [The therapist awaits feedback from the client in order to learn whether she has accepted the suggestion:] Let me know when you are sitting there with Jerry. . . .

C: That seems to be working . . . Those doors lead into the garden and I can see the terrace outside . . . Good . . . Well, now comes the meal . . . I know I can't eat . . . I ate something at home before coming because I knew I could never handle the food . . . at least not now . . . If I don't eat, there will be embarrassing inquiries . . . so there goes the tightening feeling again. . . .

T: Whether you eat or not isn't a big deal this time . . . [The therapist again invites the client to take control by thinking of a management strategy:] How could you convey the impression of eating and eat practically nothing?

C: I guess I've managed this before . . . I can make a big deal out of cutting up the vegetables . . . then trimming all the fat away from the meat . . . and stirring up the salad . . . and searching for just the right bit of someting to put on my fork . . . My plate really looks used now, and everything is stirred around and no one could tell that it hasn't been eaten from unless they were really checking on me . . . I feel safe enough to talk a little . . . Maybe some other time I can even eat a little. . . .

The therapist and client continue in this manner, stepwise, through the dinner, the ceremonies after the dinner, the dancing, and then the preparations to leave.

T: Now it's time to go home. . . .

C: I don't think that I'm ready to try going home in someone else's car . . . I'll let Jerry drive . . . I know he'll stop and change places with me any time I ask him. . . .

T: Very good . . . You have found there were many options at different times . . . and you need time to assimilate all the ways in which your private space can continue to expand . . . and you also see that you can say "no" when that is your judgment. . . .

See yourself at home . . . very relaxed . . . and review each of the situations that came up this evening . . . each of the decisions you made . . . how aware you were that you were never trapped or in danger of collapse . . . only that you needed to look for choices . . . Now take a very deep breath . . . Leave this very helpful exploration of the future . . . let the air out . . . and watch the time clock reverse itself, the hand move backward . . . until you are right back in the present . . . When you are ready . . . give yourself the signal to move from trance consciousness to full alertness. . . .

In this future-time hypnotherapeutic demonstration, a strong emphasis was placed upon the opening up of choices, the availability of alternatives. There was a strong need in this client not to feel trapped, to have the freedom to leave the situation, to have her inner space expand. The therapist was quite active in the early part of the procedure, offering structured alternatives for action. Later, there was a shift from the therapist's finding alternatives for the client toward the client's finding her own alternatives.

During subsequent trance-consciousness sessions, the client experimented with inserting herself into a fair number of situations that were already under way. Each time, she brought up all kinds of unexpected difficulties that might arise and with which she would have to cope. Gradually she was able to venture into situations where she began with the "beginning"—that is, with making the decision to go into the situation and allowing an interval for anticipation. The "leap into the future" had repeatedly affirmed that she could deal with an event once it was ongoing, but that a critical part of the difficulty arose during the time period between the decision and the actual happening. That is, the aniticipated anxiety was worse than the event itself.

Once the client is willing to project the expectation of improved functioning into the future, then the exact point for projecting the self into the future event can be flexible. The fantasied self-in-situation begins where the client feels able to tolerate some degree of risk taking. Thus, in the example given above, it could just as well have begun when the dining-out episode had almost ended as it could have at any time earlier in the event. The psychotherapeutic value lies in the fact that the client is ready to enter at some point into an area previously burdened with anxiety and avoidance. How rapidly the client moves to the beginning of the event depends on the cues garnered from the client's experiences and behaviors.

SUBJECTIVE-TIME DISTORTION

It is paradoxical that the golden moments of pleasure, joy, and exhilaration seem to fly by as on wings of light. All too short are the vacation, the hedonistic high—certainly the subjective time of these events seems condensed. Yet, when it would have been such a relief to have the time pass quickly, as when there is pain, fearful anticipation, or unhappy depression that drags on through the night, the hands of the clock seem to have forgotten how to move, and the subjective time is so much greater than the elapsed world time.

It is not just a matter of variation of psychophysiological arousal that leads to a misperception of the passage of time, for the levels of arousal may be just as great in anxiety as in exhilaration, yet the experienced time sense may be very disparate. The Ericksons' utilization of time distortion during hypnosis showed how changes in subjective time could be applied to the management of pain and stress.[1]

Reducing Stress via Subjective-Time Expansion: Example of an Obsession

Sometimes it is possible to reduce the actual amount of world time spent ruminating about disturbed thoughts and feelings by having the client rapidly experience them while in the trance state of consciousness. In the following example, subjective time was expanded so that one minute of clock time was experienced as nine or ten minutes.

The client was a successful businessman in his middle 40s whose obsessional thinking had become more and more disabling because of the amount of time it consumed each day. He had previously had eight years of psychotherapy with another therapist and knew the possible dynamics that might be involved, but his behavior remained disabling. There had also been an experience with aversive conditioning with aggravation of the obsessional rituals. He had a "gallery of horrors" that he would have to review in detail in order to be able to leave home, to remain at work, to start back home, and so on. The horrors were composed of newspaper stories and photographs of vicious violence. The gallery review lasted about 45 minutes each time, occurred five or more times a day, and exhausted the client's physical and psychological energy. His physical health was good, and he had been referred for hypnotherapy.

Ideally, it would have been most desirable for the client to have become free of his obsession. When he came for hypnotherapy, however, it became clear that he was not ready to give up his ritualistic reviews, despite his previous psychotherapeutic and aversive conditioning experiences. Instead of attempting to eliminate his ritualistic reviews completely, therefore, the plan evolved to reduce the real-world time that would be consumed by them. In this way, the obsession could become far less disabling. The client had learned about

1. M. H. Erickson and E. M. Erickson. Further Considerations of Time Distortion: Subjective Time Condensation as Distinct from Subjective Time Expansion. *American Journal of Clinical Hypnosis*, 1958, Vol. 1, No. 2, 83–88.

and experienced trance induction and enchancement in previous sessions.

THERAPIST: [To client in waking state:] As you describe your experience, your gallery reviews have become so time-consuming that they are seriously reducing the amount of time you have left for your family, your work, and your golf game. Yesterday you left your home at eight a.m. but did not get to your office until 10:15 because you had to stop twice to go through your review rituals. That was almost ninety minutes. The first time was right after that woman with the baby on her back started to cross in front of you after the light had changed but you had hardly begun to move, and the second time was after the ambulance with the sirens going full blast passed your car. You went through the complete gallery even though you fully understood why you had the reaction.

Your fingers responded yesterday that you were not sure that you were ready to close off this gallery review. [The therapist seeks permission to proceed:] Let's ask the inner part of your mind a different kind of question. If you were able to experience the same intensity of feeling in a five-minute period, which now is spread over forty-five minutes, would that be acceptable? Into a maximum of five minutes you would condense all that discomfort, and when that episode was over, you would have more free time for yourself . . . Your right index finger gave a very strong positive response . . . Good, the inner part of your mind seems to know that you would be able to handle all that intensity in the shorter time period . . .

[The therapist mentions an earlier, difficult experience that will soon be introduced into the hypnotherapy plan:] I know that it is a very wearying experience for you to have to go through your gallery review once it is triggered off by something you hear, see, or experience in your daily life. It does seem to become more aggravated under conditions of stress, as it did last week when your father was hospitalized because of his bleeding stomach ulcer. The first time that you had to visit you father's hospital room, you had to pass the fire box in the hallway with the red axe in it and could not proceed for another forty-five minutes until the total review was completed.

[The therapist prepares the client, while still in the waking state, for the treatment plan:] In a few moments, I am going to ask you to quite deliberately trigger off a complete gallery review of horror.

However this time, two important differences will be present. First, your total experience of time will change. You know how quickly time passes during a vacation, and yet the same world time may seem so much longer when you are expecting a telephone call. During your gallery reveiw, I shall be counting from FIFTEEN to ONE, and each count will feel like the passage of three minutes of subjective time. All your usual gallery review experiences will occur with the same emotional intensity, but they will be condensed into a maximum of five minutes of actual time. Eventually, as you practice with this method, you may require less than five minutes of clock time, or you may have a complete discharge of tension by the time you reach the count of EIGHT or SEVEN.

As for the second difference, you know that there are many things you remember every day and others that you forget. Sometimes you purposefully put things aside; other times you are not even aware that you have put things aside and lost them from your memory . . . Some things you tag for remembering . . . other things for forgetting. . . .

[The therapist seeks the client's permission to proceed:] I am going to ask the inner part of your mind if it would be appropriate for you to begin putting into the "forgotton storage bank," right after you have gone through your gallery review, some small or big part of the gallery review. Also, after the episode is over, I am going to ask that you experience a very profound sense of relief, as if more of the tension is being discharged each time and it will take much longer to rebuild . . . Your right index finger came up very promptly and strongly. . . .

[The therapist summarizes the agreed-upon course of events:] So it will be all right for you to go through your gallery review; for you to experience it within the total count from FIFTEEN to ONE: for you to store a bit of the review from time to time in the "forgotten bank," and for you to experience a deep sense of relief when the episode is over.

[The therapist instructs the client to put himself in trance:] Give yourself the signal with your right hand on your left shoulder and then deepen your trance as you have learned.

[The therapist suggests two levels of functioning:] Throughout this experience, I am going to ask the conscious part of you to remain with me, while the inner part of your mind takes you to the lobby of the hospital waiting room by the elevator door. It is early in the morning and not many visitors are here. . . .

[The therapist paces the process, seeking feedback from the client:] When you see yourself as ready to push the elevator button to call the elevator, please signal with your right index finger . . . Good. . . .

Now enter the elevator and go up to the fifth floor. Turn to the right as you leave the elevator and wave your hand to the nurse who takes care of your father as you pass the nurse's station. Now move on down into Corridor D until you come to where the fire box with the red-handled fireaxe is located. [Again, the therapist seeks feedback:] When you reach that place, lift your right index finger. . . .

I shall begin to count from FIFTEEN to ONE. When I reach ONE, your total full review will be over; you will take two very deep breaths, and release them. When that is over, you will feel very light . . . quiet, detached . . . very comfortable, with a sense of relief . . . with your tensions fully discharged, and you may even wonder why you had been so tense in the first place. . . .

FIFTEEN . . . FOURTEEN . . . THIRTEEN . . . TWELVE . . . ELEVEN . . . TEN . . . NINE . . . the review is almost half over . . . EIGHT. . . SEVEN . . . SIX . . . FIVE . . . coming to the end of the review . . . soon all the tension will be gone. . . .

[The therapist introduces the "forgotten bank":] The review will slip into the bank of forgotten memories . . . [The therapist invites the client's control:] You may forget a small bit or a larger bit . . . FOUR . . . THREE . . . TWO . . . ONE. . . .

Take a deep breath and let it out slowly . . . very good . . . Now take a second breath . . . Expand your chest fully and as it relaxes, relax all over, feel yourself drifting into a dressy state . . . The past few minutes seem so far away, and there is so much free space in front of you to enjoy and look forward to . . . Give yourself the signal to arouse yourself and to feel alert, relaxed, and unusually free of tension . . .

The client was visibly agitated and stressed during his horror review. He clenched his fists, gritted his teeth, perspired profusely, and breathed heavily. If he had been hooked up to a recording machine, it is reasonably certain that a much accelerated heartbeat would have been recorded. However, by the time that the count of

FIVE was given, there were indications of decreased tension. When he opened his eyes, he appeared calm and actually relaxed.

T: [To the client, who has aroused himself from the trance:] You went through a very difficult stress experience, but now you have freed up more time. You condensed the suffering into a much shorter period of actual time, and you will very likely be free of your obsessional thoughts for a much longer period of time because of the deeper discharge of inner tensions.

The client was not willing to repeat the experience at that session, but on the next visit he reported that he had practiced the exercise each morning before leaving home, and in the office before leaving for the hospital to visit his father. The frequency of the episodes had dropped to three a day, and he had managed with a maximum of eight to ten actual minutes per episode. He was most impressed with the relief that he felt after each episode, explaining that "it was as if a heavy burden was laid aside for a while. When it comes back I don't try to fight it. I just find a place, relax, and go through the count." The reviews were repeated during the next four sessions.

Therapeutic sessions were continued over the six-month period but were not focused upon the obsessional problems. In a follow-up visit four years later, the client reported that he had coped reasonably well with his father's death, and had expanded his business and personal life considerably. He still took about 10–15 minutes of each day to do his "review exercises," but was very reluctant to disturb what he considered an adequate equilibrium.

Reducing Stress via Subjective-Time Condensation

There are life situations where world time cannot be decreased, but where accessibility to a contracted or condensed subjective-time experience would provide the client with considerable relief. While in trance, the client learns, for example, how to experience ten minutes of clock time as five minutes, then as one minute, and ultimately even as one second. Under these conditions, the client may experience traveling through the stress situation at a far more rapid subjective pace than the elapsed world time. Sometimes the client will report that the wall clock is moving in peculiar, jumpy fashion: The minute hand may jump in quarter-hour units, or move more like the second hand. People may be seen as moving about rapidly; there may be amnesic gaps. As one client reported: "The nurse came in, started an IV . . . went out and came right in and started another IV . . . This was funny, because before it was always a couple of hours between IV's but this felt like only a few minutes . . . The day was over before I noticed it. . . ."

Condensation of subjective time may make it easier for the client to cope with critical periods involving heightened pain and stress that have a considerable world-time duration. The subjectively condensed time makes the situation more tolerable, especially when it is coupled with subjectively expanded time during periods of relatively low stress or pain. During the hypnotherapeutic trance, the client is also supported by suggestions for recovery of energy, for body mobilization, for healing, and for rapid fading from memory of the stressful experience that is now over.

The hypnotherapeutic expansion or condensation of subjective time draws on imagery relevant to the particular client in the given treatment situation. It is used, whenever feasible, in conjunction with other approaches to reducing stress. However, there may be times when the client's confidence is so depleted, or when the personal significance of the distrubance is such, that subjective-time distortion is the most accessible approach for easing the passage through pain. The therapist must be ready to persist in supporting the client in the mode of managing the distress, since a real therapeutic gain may not become manifest until several collaborative "passages" have been conducted with the client.

The ability of clients to engage in some form of dissociation by adopting dual levels of functioning at the same time was used to advantage in some of the cases presented in this and preceding chapters. The following chapter elaborates dissociation as a hypnotherapeutic tool.

Dissociation

"Dissociation" generally refers to a state in which a group of mental processes have become separated from other mental processes with which they are ordinarily associated. Examples are cases of double and multiple personality, delusions, fugue states, conversion paralysis, and the more commonly experienced everyday trance states (see pp. 12–13).

The capacity of an individual to act as an observer of his or her own behavior in ordinary life, and in this way to separate or dissociate that self from the self in the situation, is a fairly universal ability. The student who is called upon to talk before a class may experience part of the self as speaking to the audience, yet may be aware of another part of the self functioning as observer, watching the performing self and wondering if the verbal presentation is up to standard. The individual is both detached as observer and actively engaged as performer. The process of acting in a play is another illustration: The performer-self is immersed in portraying the character in the play while the observer-self assesses and guides the presentation of the acted role. Awareness exists of the separation of the two spheres of functioning, as well as of the capability of merging them as needed.

The competency of the individual to move between separation and integration may become impaired or totally dysfunctional—that is, unresponsive to intentional decision or situational demand. Such a disruption would interfere with the capacity to test reality, and may be a significant aspect of serious personality disorders.

Dissociation can be utilized during hypnotherapy to help the person separate a part of the self from the self that is experiencing a particular situation, because the separated part can then become reintegrated as needed.

ASPECTS OF HYPNOTIC DISSOCIATION

Almost all individuals who experience hypnotic states of consciousness describe their awareness of self during trance in such terms as these: "I was detached," "I was feeling that it was myself but a somewhat different me," "I was feeling freer, less constrained," or "There seemed to be a part of me that I was experiencing that was not usually in my awareness." This type of descriptive language occurs so regularly and so spontaneously that it seems reasonable to state that there is a tendency to experience some kind of "distancing" between the experience of self in the usual waking state of consciousness and the experience of self in the hypnotic state of consciousness.

It may well be that in the hypnotic state of consciousness, useful aspects of dissociated states can become more readily available than in the waking state. For example, the careful work of the Hilgards on the experience of pain during hypnosis strongly suggests the existence of a "hidden observer" within the self that functions to record aspects of an ongoing experience that are withheld from awareness.[1] Under certain conditions, the "hidden observer" can become available not only to the self in hypnosis, but also to the self in waking consciousness. These observations, along with many others, support the conclusion that some type of dissociative experience is characteristic of the hypnotic state of consciousness.

Three dimensions or aspects of the dissociative experience can be distinguished: (1) detachment (the awareness of a distancing of the waking self from the self in hypnotic consciousness); (2) altered self-control (the experience that some parts of the self have a tendency to become more autonomous, or free from the usual constraints of the waking state); and (3) selective awareness (the experience that some aspects of the self in hypnosis are amenable to amnesia or other processes of selective withholding from the waking consciousness).

If these three dimensions are reasonably separate aspects of the dissociative experience of self during hypnosis, then some interesting inferences or speculations become possible. For example, the analgesic experience of hypnoanesthesia might well be considerably enhanced through the extension of the detachment aspect of the dissociative experience. With respect to altered self-control, it may well be that some conditions of intense anxiety of rapid onset in the waking state tend to induce a "spontaneous" state of hypnosis in which the individual is disposed to suggest to the self the idea of decreased self-control. In such instances, the hypnotherapeutic intervention might well be to help the client experience an increasing sense of control over the

1. E. R. Hilgard and J. R. Hilgard. *Hypnosis in the Relief of Pain*. Los Altos, California: Kaufmann, 1975.

mounting anxiety. As for selective awareness, insofar as the hypnotic state of consciousness can result in a *complete* separation between the awareness of self in trance from the awareness of self in the awake state, then understanding fugue states and multiple personalities as instances of extended trance states becomes a credible possibility.

It should be noted that dissociation, in the broadest sense of the term, is involved in all hypnotherapeutic procedures. A more explicit focus on dissociation as such can also be incorporated in these procedures—for example, in age retrogression, guided imagery, and projection. A case in point is the demonstration of age retrogression with the "don't cry" procedure (Chapter 6, pp. 86–90), in which the client experienced dual levels of functioning: vividly "reliving" a past event while maintaining an observer–interpreter stance.

The remainder of the present chapter describes three different uses of hypnotic dissociation and the disparate purposes for which they are invoked. In the first two of these (finger signaling and dissociative writing and drawing), the aim is to reduce conscious control over the performing self as far as possible. In the third case—namely, coexistent selves as observer and participant—the intent is to create an emotional distance between the two parts of the self while at the same time enabling the person to remain aware of what is occurring in the actual situation.

FINGER SIGNALING

Clinically, finger signaling is probably the most frequent use of the dissociative experience in hypnosis. The procedure for the establishment of finger signals has already been presented in Chapter 2.

To briefly summarize the procedure: The client is reminded that there is an "inner part of the mind" wherein much awareness, experience, feeling, information, and capacity for judgment are stored. This knowledge can be of considerable value to the individual in the decision- and action-making process. The "inner part of the mind" influences the individual's behavior whether or not the individual is aware of it. However, if the individual is able to bridge the communication gap between the "up-front" part of his or her mind and the "inner part of the mind," then there can be greater confidence in the decision or action. One method that has been found useful in bridging this gap is asking the client to suspend "voluntary intention" in the moving of his or her fingers. Instead, "involuntary movement" by the inner part of the mind is encouraged according to a prearranged system of finger signaling (see pp. 29–31).

The therapist's instructions, explanation, and suggestions concerning finger signaling are directed toward optimal utilization of the dissociative aspect of the hypnotic experience. Through the finger-signaling mode of communication, an alternative to the voluntary response becomes possible for the purpose of facilitating the expression of ambivalence. The involuntary finger movements, through the intervention of the inner part of the mind, indicate altered self-control. Time and again, clients are surprised by the discrepancy between their verbal (conscious-control) response and the finger-signaling response. Where there is consonance between the verbal response and the finger response, the client may have greater confidence in the verbal decision and a greater commitment to the suggested action.

Moreover, the signaling procedure, when used as an integral part of the therapy to elicit the client's guidance about direction, content, and action, strongly involves the client in comanaging the therapeutic process. Of course, there are structural limitations to any inquiry where the response possibilities are limited to "yes," "no," "I don't know," and "I do not choose to answer."

Although the initiative for the finger-signaling inquiry and the probing questions typically come from the therapist, there is no reason why the client may not also learn to function as the initiator of inquiries, as well as the formulator of questions to the self.

AUTOMATIC WRITING AND DRAWING: EXAMPLE OF DISSOCIATIVE IMAGERY

Automatic writing and drawing procedures are designed to elicit responses from the inner part of the mind that are not limited to the four categories of the finger-signaling responses. However, effective responsiveness to dissociative writing or drawing procedures takes a much longer period of training on the part of the client. A smaller proportion of clients than in the case of finger signaling become sufficiently productive with these procedures to warrant their use early in the hypnotherapeutic experience. The difficulty may be a function of the complexity of the dissociative process, or may be related to the particular automatic-writing dissociative procedure described below. In my clinical practice, these procedures are considered as a potential resource when other hypnotherapeutic methods have been quite unproductive.

Although the following procedure refers specifically to automatic writing, the procedure can readily be modified to apply to automatic drawing as well. One would then refer to the "drawing hand" instead of the "writing hand," or suggest that the inner part of the mind move the hand "to begin drawing" instead of "to begin writing," and so forth.

The client is given a clipboard with a supply of blank sheets numbered from 1 to 25, along with a felt-tipped pen for easy writing with a minimum of pressure. The clipboard is used because it can be placed in the client's lap with the writing hand holding the pen relaxed upon it, a position not often used by most people when writing. Typically the eyes of the client are closed, although some people readily write without conscious control while keeping their eyes open. Some clinicians have advocated suspending the writing arm in a sling to facilitate free movement.

The client in the following example had had experience with self-induction and enhancement of the trance state in previous sessions.

THERAPIST: [To client in waking state:] You know how helpful it has been thus far to have the use of finger signals to tap into the way your inner mind has felt about many of the things that have come up thus far . . . It has become important to know even further about some of the inner things that may be going on within you that are contributing to your present level of stress . . . The inner part of your mind, the inner self, may know a great deal about this that may be helpful to you if we knew more about the questions to ask that could enable this understanding to become available to your waking mind . . . [The therapist seeks permission to proceed:] Before we begin, let us check with the inner part of your mind whether it would be okay to use automatic writing [or drawing] as a way to tell us what would help your treatment to progress . . . Your right index finger has signaled that this would be acceptable. . . .

Place this pen in your writing hand in your usual writing position, and place your hand on the clipboard in your lap. There are many sheets of blank paper on the clipboard. From time to time, as may be necessary, I will remove the top sheet so that you will always have plenty of clean writing surface . . . Make yourself comfortable and let your writing arm relax very completely onto the clipboard on your lap . . . [The therapist begins making dissociative suggestions:] You are going to put your writing hand into good connection with the inner part of your mind after you have temporarily disconnected it from your conscious mind . . . As the connection with the inner part of your mind becomes stronger and stronger, you will find yourself less and less aware of what your writing arm and hand are doing . . . which gives the inner part of your mind a better chance to communicate through your writing hand . . . .

Take a deep breath . . . Hold it in and very slowly let the air come out . . . [The therapist offers concrete imagery leading to the dimming of a light bulb, to be used in the process of dissociation:] As you feel the air moving out of your chest, let yourself feel that your writing arm is becoming light and transparent, as if you could see inside your arm and see the nerves that look like wiring connecting it to your active, controlling part of you brain . . . Visualize the wiring ending up in a light in the controlling part of your brain . . . [The therapist suggests gradual, not sudden, dissociation:] As the connection between your writing hand and the controlling part of your conscious mind diminishes, notice how the light becomes dimmer and dimmer . . . Your writing hand may begin to feel somewhat cooler . . . even a bit on the numb side, and there may be a gradual decrease of all sense of heaviness in your hand and arm and even up to the shoulder, where the inner wiring crosses over into the neck and head . . . Soon almost all the up-front control will be turned off and you will notice that the light is almost completely turned off; just the barest glow remains . . . [The therapist seeks guidance from the client:] When the light has reached that point, nod your head . . . Feel that detached, even floating experience in your writing hand . . . how far away and separate from your conscious-control mind it feels . . . Even the sensations from the fingers holding the pen are fading away . . . but the pen remains held in position . . . The sensations of the clipboard against your hand become dim and distant. . . .

[The suggestions strengthen the connection with the inner mind:] Soon you will begin to experience the awareness of a different light coming from the *inner* part of your mind . . . from that inner self. As the light increases . . . begin to feel a different sort of connection in your writing arm and hand . . . as if there was a gentle warmth and aliveness coming into the shoulder, the arm, the hand, and the fingers . . . You can see a different set of wires beginning to pulse with action, and the arm, hand, and shoulder become less and less transparent . . . The feeling becomes stronger and stronger as the light increases the connection between the inner part of your mind and the writing hand . . . It is as if the hand has a life of its own and there is an impulse for the hand and the pen to begin moving, to begin writing, yet the conscious part of your mind is not aware of what is being written. . . .

Let the inner part of your mind feel free to communicate whatever is most significant at this time about your difficulties . . . [A second activity is introduced to encourage automatic writing:] While this is going on, we can discuss our last session . . . Your hand will continue with its writing without being distracted by our discussion . . . [The therapist offers a nonverbal way to indicate the end of the writing:] When the messages from the inner part of your mind are completed, your writing hand will release the pen, and your hand will open up and come to rest on the clipboard with the palm facing upward. . . .

[The therapist then involves the client in a therapeutically relevant discussion, until the pen-drop signal is given that the messages have been completed.]

Good, your hand has signaled that the messages have been transmitted for the present . . . [The therapist introduces the process of restoring normal control:] Now begin to have that special warm and detached feeling in your hand, arm, and shoulder begin to diminish . . . And the connections between your writing hand and the inner part of your mind begin to fade . . . Notice how the previous process begins to reverse itself . . . The light with that special quality in the inner part of your mind is beginning to decrease in intensity, and as the special light fades, the light in your conscious-control center begins to increase in intensity. The nerve network comes back into action . . . The normal feelings, sensations, and weight are returning to your writing hand, your wrist, your forearm, your shoulder . . . and as it returns, the coolness and the numbness disappear. . . .

[The therapist uses number progression to maintain the trance while restoring proper control connections:] In a moment, I shall ask you to take a deep breath . . . to hold it, and then to let it out slowly while I count from FIVE to ONE . . . When I reach ONE, you will have had all the time you need to restore all the connections that allow conscious control of your arm, as well as the connections to that part of your inner mind that functions with the finger signals . . . FIVE . . . FOUR . . . THREE . . . The connections are almost completed . . . TWO . . . ONE . . . Your hand, arm, and shoulder are comfortably reconnected. . . .

[The therapist encourages translatability of the automatic writing:] You can let yourself remain in trance while you open your eyes to examine what your inner mind wrote by means of your writing hand . . . Your conscious mind will be able to translate what your hand has written . . . The meaning will gradually become clear not only while you are in trance but in the waking state as well . . . Let your eyes open when you are ready. . . .

Some of the problems with automatic writing arise from the form of the products. The writing may be scrawled. Letters may be only partially formed. There may be mirror writing. The writing may wander all over the page, criss-crossing paths. In addition to the cryptographic elements, there may be symbol substitutions—for example, "B-4" for "before." With practice, however, there is some improvement of legibility, and the method holds considerable promise for a few clients. More often, the product becomes a basis for "projective" translation rather than for dissociative interpretation.

COEXISTENT SELVES AS OBSERVER AND PARTICIPANT: EXAMPLE OF BURN-DRESSING CHANGE

The kind of psychological dissociation that allows a person to distance himself or herself emotionally from actually occurring ongoing events can be achieved in a variety of ways during trance. The case to be presented is one specific illustration of a promising procedure. It is important to note that the dissociative process revealed in the example is linked with the integrative process as two aspects of the experience. Notice also that the client was encouraged to introduce variants into the dissociative process that would sustain the continued effectiveness of the procedure.

In the following demonstration, guided imagery was extensively used in the dissociative process. The client was a woman in her mid-30s who had suffered severe burns on her left thigh and leg when a kettle filled with scalding water had slipped from her hands. Her pain was relatively well managed except for the times when dressings had to be changed. There was considerable concern on the part of her physician because of the increasing doses of analgesic drugs that became necessary during these periods.

The client had had previous experience with hypnosis as a subject in an experiment, and therefore her physician suggested the possibility of hypnoanalgesia. An eager participant, she showed considerable capacity to enter into trance and use trance phenomena. She quickly learned to use subjective-time condensation as a method of making time pass more quickly in the hospital (see Chapter 6, pp. 104–105). She also revealed that she was an avid gardener, and that her accident had been related to some of her canning work. She was encouraged to describe some of her gardening interests in detail.

THERAPIST: [In hospital room] Janice, both you and your doctor have expressed concern about the amount of pain medication you have had to use in order to tolerate the stress of the dressing changes. You are familiar with hypnotic trance and are quite competent in maintaining a trance. [The therapist seeks confirmation after giving instruction in finger signaling:] I would like to ask the inner part of your mind if it would be in the best interest for your healing if you were able to reduce the amount of these analgestic medications . . . And your right index finger very promptly answered "yes" . . . No hesitation there . . . There is a special type of experience you could have with the use of your hypnotic trance, which would markedly decrease, if not entirely eliminate, your need for medication during the particularly stressful experience of having your dressing changed. [The therapist seeks further confirmation:] Would the inner part of your mind be comfortable with your leaving your physical body behind in this room while you and I took a walk in your garden?

CLIENT: You mean that you and I would leave here and go to my garden while I left my physical body here for them to treat my left leg and thigh? I'm not sure I fully grasp what you are saying.

T: [The therapist clarifies by offering an analogy:] Did you ever have to give a talk before a group? Do you remember that when you got up in front of the group to talk, you felt as though only part of you was standing up in front of the group, and that the rest of you was somewhere "out there" watching yourself give the talk?

C: Yes. That's true.

T: Wasn't that an interesting experience? . . . You were one person all the time, but part of you could be giving a speech and another part of you could be watching yourself give the speech, wondering what was going to be coming out next, and feeling detached and separated from the part of you that was talking and doing a job in front of the group.

This kind of ability can be very helpful as a way to increase your ability to cope with pain. You know, in your fantasy, it is possible for you to close your eyes and imagine that you are in the mountains or at the seaside, and the scene can become more real than what is going on here in the room. [The therapist again seeks permission to proceed:] Let's ask your inner mind if it is acceptable for us to venture on that path . . . Give yourself the cue to go into trance, and when you are well into your trance, have your inner mind review the issue and signal by either the "yes" or "no" index finger. [The client's right index finger for "yes" rises almost immediately.]

Very good . . . Take a deep breath . . . Hold it for the count of five . . . Now let the air move out very slowly . . . quietly . . . feel it move out through your nose . . . As it moves out . . . let the tension in the chest flow out down your arms . . . into the bed frame . . . down the bed frame into the floor and then into the earth . . . letting go as profoundly as you have ever been able to do in the past . . . perhaps even more completely than ever before . . . As you reach the right level of letting go for yourself . . . imagine yourself as getting up from where you are and coming over to where I am . . . Let your right index finger come up when you see yourself as being near me and also can observe yourself lying quietly in bed . . . Tell me how you feel. . . .

C: A little bit funny . . . The part of me lying down looks somewhat more solid and substantial . . . I can feel myself near you but can't see myself there as yet . . . However, I do feel myself as being both in my body and outside of my body . . . As I'm talking, I am beginning to imagine and see myself near you, but there seems to be a third part of me observing the other two. . . .

T: That's fine . . . That is often the experience as you begin working with the process . . . In just a while the sense of the third position will fade . . . when you are ready . . . and the observer "you" will become much more definite . . . Okay. Now let us leave Janice lying in her bed and let us take seats on the other side of the room near the door. The physical Janice, with her injured body, will remain comfortable on the bed, while the inner part of you, the part full of creative imagery, will move to the other side of the room. [The therapist invites the client's active participation:] Which chair will you take?

C: [While in trance] I think I will take the straight-backed chair. . . .

T: Fine . . . I'll take the one with the arms. Janice, look toward the bed and tell me what the scene is. . . .

C: I see Janice in her yellow bed jacket lying in the bed and looking out of the window. There is the apparatus over her left leg and thigh to keep her foot clear of contact with the covers. I can see a light shining through the sheets. Janice has a book open, but she is not really reading. Her eyelids seem to be getting very heavy and she is feeling quite drowsy. Her hair looks like it needs tidying up—it hasn't had any real attention since the accident. The grey is beginning to show through, and that isn't so good for her vanity.

T: [The therapist supports the client's progress:] It is good that you are noticing Janice's hair, because until just a short while ago Janice was so overwhelmed by her left thigh and leg that she didn't have time to notice the comforting, everyday things she used to do. You are right, Janice does look very relaxed and almost ready to doze off. The doctor and his nurse should be along soon to change Janice's dressing, so we might as well be out of their way while they are busy. The marvelous part of the magic we are sharing is that we can walk down to the end of the hospital corridor, go through the exit doors, and be right in your garden. Shall we start?

C: What if Janice should need me?

T: There is no reason why you can't be in touch with her if she should need you. Her thoughts can become part of your awareness, and you can comfort her and transmit your support to her no matter where you are. Janice's physical self will be getting the proper treatment with the change of dressing, and you will be able to transmit comforting thoughts to her if necessary. At the same time you will be enjoying your trip through the garden, showing me the many things you have worked so hard to develop. . . .

The client seemed quite reassured with this, and the next 45 minutes were spent by Janice and her therapist in the imagined garden. She described the varieties of flowers and her plan for the planting of bulbs in the fall. At about 10 minutes into the "garden trip," the burn team arrived to change the dressing and was finished in about 20 minutes. Twice during the procedure, the client very vigorously and strongly clasped the hand of the therapist and said, intensely, "Janice is feeling distressed." The therapist, guiding the healing process, replied, "Send your full comfort and support to her. Tell her to shut off all feeling to the leg and thigh and let her full energy go into the healing. It seems to be coming along fine. We can go back if she really needs us. I think that she feels good about our being in the garden." In less than 15 seconds, the client had resumed her discussion of the garden.

After the burn team left, the therapist said:

T: Our time is almost finished for today, so let's return to the hospital room. When you are outside the hospital door, raise your right index finger . . . Good . . . Open the door quietly because Janice is very relaxed and resting. I will sit in my chair and you cross the room and fuse together with Janice, who is feeling so good about how well she handled the treatment procedure today. In a little while I shall count from ONE to FIVE. When I reach FIVE, let your eyes open gently and feel positive all over. ONE . . . TWO . . . THREE . . . arousing yourself . . . FOUR . . . almost awake . . . FIVE . . . completely awake and remembering your visit to your garden with pleasure. . . .

The client and therapist repeated the training sessions each day for the next four days, then on alternative days for a week, and finally in one practice–reinforcement session per week until the client left the hospital.

The examples presented in this chapter illustrate how hypnosis can be used for therapeutic purposes to help the client separate parts of the self that are ordinarily connected. In the case of finger signaling and of automatic writing or drawing, the separation of the motoric system from conscious control provided a new medium for relaying unconscious thoughts and feelings. The example of the dual roles of the self as both observer and participant served a different purpose, that of pain control.

Observer–participant separation can also serve other purposes. Actually, whenever a client describes what is happening in an imaged scene in which he or she is participating, it can be said that dissociation in the form of coexisting selves as observer and participant has occurred. Examples of this form of dissociation can be found throughout this volume. The purposes are varied: to gain understanding, to release feelings, to relieve anxiety, to control pain, and to image and practice new ways of reacting or behaving in general.

Role Reversal and Induced Conflict

Two additional hypnotherapeutic procedures that can be used by psychotherapists of varying persuasions are client–therapist role reversal and induced conflict. It is assumed that the client has already been involved in the therapeutic relationship beyond the initial assessment phase, and that the client has achieved some competence in the use of hypnosis.

CLIENT–THERAPIST ROLE REVERSAL: EXAMPLE OF CLIENT INDECISIVENESS

In client–therapist role reversal, the client and therapist assume each other's roles while the client is in the state of trance consciousness. Although it is not necessary for the client to have achieved a good level of competence in utilizing hypnosis, such competence clearly helps. Shifting roles is easier for clients who are able comfortably to initiate thoughts and action while in trance. Sometimes it is helpful to shift roles back and forth several times as the encounter develops.

The role-reversal procedure is often useful when the therapist has become unclear about the direction the therapeutic process might take, or when the client has reached an impasse in coping with a given situation. Clinicians have also found that the procedure can be helpful when it is important for a client to become more clearly aware of the progress that has already been made in therapy. When this is the purpose, the client in the role of therapist is encouraged to affirm the changes that have occurred during the course of therapy by pointing them out to the therapist, who, for the time being, has assumed the role of client.

The case illustration to follow indicates how the client–therapist role reversal procedure helped the client through a crisis of vacillation when he was required to make an important professional career decision. The client was a 42-year-old married man with three teenage children. Six months earlier, substantial pressures at work precipitated a strong anxiety reaction with marked gastrointestinal concomitants. During the course of psychotherapy, the client learned how to use hypnotherapeutic techniques to relax, to interrupt the escalation of tension, to distance himself from problems when he needed perspective, and to re-educate his physiology through appropriate outward release of anger. His somatic reactions became significantly milder, and his occasional depressive episodes were reduced in intensity and duration. Then came an offer for a position in a new setting, with an increase of salary and much better potential for his particular work. The time limit for accepting the position was rapidly approaching. The invitation apparently had reactivated some of the old patterns of anxiety and gastrointestinal turbulence. The client had already spent three sessions agonizing over the pros and cons of the decision. The second and third sessions were almost total reproductions of the first session, with no indication that he was moving any closer to a decision.

THERAPIST: [To client in waking state:] Your decision time is next Friday. Even if you do nothing, it will still be a decision. It is clear that doing nothing is a real alternative . . . Yet, when the inner part of your mind was questioned, it expressed the preference for an active decision of acceptance or rejection of the offer . . . At the same time, the finger signals indicated that the inner part of your mind was just as undecided about the decision as your active conscious mind has been . . . Thus far, we have not been able to find a way to help you get closer to a decision. This may be a good time for us to change places . . . You have had the time to observe me closely for almost six months . . . and you know how I approach things, how I relate to you . . . But you have, in addition, knowledge about yourself that covers your whole lifetime . . . I have listened to you, have tuned in on you, and have come to know how you express things during the time we have spent together. So let's combine these resources in a new way.

In a short while I am going to ask you to put yourself into a trance state . . . and to see yourself as taking over my role as therapist . . . At the same time, I will also move over and become you, move into your role as the client . . . We will be working over this difficult decision problem . . . But you will have the combined assets of knowing about the therapist role and also being able to draw on your knowledge of yourself from all levels of your awareness of yourself . . . So you will help me, your client, find a way of reaching a decision that I can stick with about the job offer. . . .

Breathe in deeply . . . Close your eyes . . . Let the air out slowly as you move into your trance consciousness . . . Breathe in once again . . . Hold it! . . . As you breathe out, relax profoundly and go as deeply into trance as you need to in order to have optimal contact with your inner experience and be able to speak easily . . . I will count from FIVE to ONE and when I reach ONE . . . you will be profoundly, deeply, and comfortably relaxed . . . calm . . . detached . . . FIVE . . . FOUR . . . THREE . . . TWO . . . ONE . . . Quiet . . . Your body is functioning comfortably . . . a strong feeling of confidence in yourself flowing through you . . . I am going to ask your fingers whether it is okay for you to completely take over the therapist role at this time while I take over your role as client . . . The "yes" finger came up . . . Fine . . . In any way that is comfortable for you, see yourself move over into my role as therapist . . . You will be helping me to find a way of reaching a decision that I can stay with and be happy with . . . When you see yourself there . . . signal to me with your finger . . . Good. . . .

CLIENT ROLE [THERAPIST][1]: I just can't reach a decision and hold on it. There is no way out of it. I must reach a decision by next Friday. I've been over the same ground a hundred times alone and with Marylou [the client's wife]. She keeps saying that she will be completely comfortable with whatever decision I make, whether we go or we stay. In a funny way, that doesn't seem to help. I almost think that it would have been easier if I did not have psychotherapy. Then I was so unhappy here I would have given anything to get away. Now that I've learned to get on top of the job and feel good about what I have achieved, I hate to throw this success away. Even though the new job will pay better and looks like an advance for my career, there are so many unknowns in it.

THERAPIST ROLE [CLIENT]: There is no other choice for you this time. You will have to make a decision about this on your own. Neither Marylou nor I want to, or could, make this decision for you. Once you have made up your mind, then we will both know how to go on from there. Nothing has really changed about the job here. You know, in your heart, that the same conditions exist now that were present last February. You are the one who has changed. These

---

1. The bracketed identification indicates who is playing the specified role.

changes will be there whether you are here or in the new place. You want me to press you into making a decision so you can blame me for not giving you enough time or some other excuse.

C ROLE [T]: I really don't want to blame anybody. Each time I make the decision, then I begin to think of Marylou and all the friends she has made here, how well she likes the place, and how the kids are happy in the schools, and the decision becomes unglued. It fades away.

T ROLE [C]: It really bugs you that Marylou is not upset about the possible move. That she hasn't gone into high gear to push you one way or the other. If only someone important to you would take a definite stand about what you should do. It wouldn't matter what it was, but then you'd really know how to organize yourself into the opposite position, whether or not it was good for your career in the short run or the long run. It won't work this time. You are really ready to make a decision, and you can make it because Marylou said that she could live with either staying or going. She likes the changes in you and isn't afraid of how you will react after you make the decision.

C ROLE [T]: I see. You really feel that I've gone over things long enough and that nothing new is going to show up, and that Marylou and I can make either decision work out. I know that you've made the point again and again that although this is an important decision, it is not a life-and-death one, and we can always make another move in five years.

T: [The therapist returns to his own role, changes tone and tempo of his voice, and says to the client, who is still in trance:] Now we are back in our own roles . . . Take a moment . . . Breathe in deeply, hold it, and let the air out slowly and relax as I count form ONE to FIVE . . . When I reach FIVE, you will be yourself in your own wide-awake role . . . ONE . . . TWO . . . THREE . . . FOUR . . . FIVE . . . Give yourself your cue to shift from the trance state to your usual waking state, and we will discuss what just happened. . . .

The client–therapist role reversal was helpful to the client. In the posthypnotic discussion, the client made clear that the experience helped him to become clearer about how much Marylou's equanimity in the situation bothered him. He also thought that the therapist had been too permissive in not pressing him for a decision and was surprised that he felt confident that whatever decision he would make would be one that he could "live with." He decided that he would accept the new position. He was also surprised at how much irritation he showed as "therapist" toward the "client," and wondered how the therapist could tolerate so much procrastination.

Clients, in general, find the role-reversal encounter to be a rewarding experience yielding therapeutic insight into themselves. They report quite consistently that they come as a result to recognize much more clearly how important it is for them to assume an active role and take responsibility for their own therapy.

The therapist can encourage the client, even after therapy has been terminated, to make use of the role-reversal method by fantasizing the role of therapist when confronted by old or new problems. The clinical procedure can become part of a lasting practicum experience for helping the client move toward greater competence and confidence in managing problems of living without formal therapeutic assistance.

CONFLICT INDUCED DURING TRANCE: EXAMPLE OF A SECRET EATER

A psychological conflict may be induced in the individual during the trance state itself, or as a posthypnotic suggestion. In either case, the induced-conflict procedure is one that should be used judiciously, since there is always the possibility that the added stress may overload the client's ability to deal with the life situation in question, and perhaps may result in unexpected decompensating behavior.

When appropriately used, however, the induced-conflict experience may have considerable psychotherapeutic value for certain clients who are avoiding or denying important aspects of their problems. For example, the experience may be helpful for those clients who consistently cannot recognize the harmful psychological maneuvers they devise when under stress; or for clients who are reluctant to get in touch with their own feelings because of uncertainty or fear about what they will need to admit and to face. The induced conflict should be clearly related to the client's problem area so that the client can readily grasp the connection.

In the following illustration, a posthypnotic suggestion induced a conflict related to the client's eating problem. The client, an intelligent, competent professional woman in her late 30s, was much distressed by her excessive weight (42 pounds above the norms for her height). Over the past 13 years, she had gone through several cycles of big diet, big loss, and big regaining of weight. She had sampled a wide range of psychotherapeutic approaches and was conversant with most of the theories about obesity. When she came to the therapist seeking "help from hypnosis," she was not looking for a "miracle cure," but was looking for some way to develop a new pattern of eating that would put an end to her yo-yo fluctuations. She had been with this particular psychotherapist for nine weeks. During this time, she became secure and confident in utilizing trance and was able to visualize and fantasize with ease. The daily logs of food intake that were part of the eating-control plan had been faithfully kept for the previous six weeks, yet her weight loss was considerably less than the usual weight loss on such a high-protein, moderate-calorie intake. This gap had been discussed by the client and her therapist without contributing to better understanding.

The therapist wondered whether the client could be a "secret eater" who was so conflicted over her extra food intake that she had found a way to hide this intake from herself. It was the therapist's judgment that she could handle the extra stress of induced conflict, even though the conflict would touch on an area of greater personal sensitivity.

In preparation for the session, the therapist had placed two plastic bags, partially filled with M & M chocolates, on a small end table close to where the client would be seated. The client, who regularly taped her therapy sessions for later review, could also place her tape recorder and microphone on this table. When she had done so at the begining of the session, she made no overt gesture of having recognized the candy.

THERAPIST: [To the client in the waking state:] You definitely shed some weight during the past six weeks. But it is puzzling that your weight loss is so much less than expected with your following the diet plan so strictly. I would like to suggest an interesting procedure that might yield some clues toward understanding that gap. Would you be interested?

CLIENT: Of course! I simply do not understand it. [The client notices the bag of candy.] This candy looks like real temptation.

T: Those M & Ms were left behind by someone else who has no weight problem. I've left them there to be sure that she would see them and remember to pick them up this afternoon. If I put them in my desk they would just be forgotten. . . .

Why don't you push yourself back in the chair until you are comfortable? . . . [The therapist invites trance-induction procedure that the client has practiced:] Give yourself your signal to begin moving into the trance state . . . [The therapist refers to the customary procedure for this client:] Let your eyes move way up as if you were looking through the crown of your head . . . When your eyelids begin to feel real fluttery . . . your right arm will float up into the air as if it were attached to a marvelous balloon filled with helium . . . just the way it usually does when you let yourself relax . . . Relax all over . . . Let every part of you let go so fully that it feels like you are opening up an especially good connection into your innermost self . . . When you reach that fullness of relaxation . . . the helium will be released slowly from the balloon and your arm will float downward into your lap . . . gently . . . Your feeling is so detached . . . so much into your own private space. . . .

Earlier, before your trance, you noticed those delicious M & M candies—how tempting they could be. You learned that they belonged to another client . . . and you know that these chocolates are definitely not part of your high-protein diet plan. . . .

[The therapist induces posthypnotic conflict:] In a little while, after you terminate your trance and are awake, you will begin to experience an ever-increasing desire to eat those candies . . . yet part of you will remain aware that they do not belong to you and that your diet prohibits eating candy. [The therapist offers the client the choice of amnesia:] You may or may not remember that this was told to you during the trance. That is something that the inner part of your mind will decide. This conflict between wanting to eat the candy and the reasons not to eat them will continue to grow strong with each passing moment . . . stronger and stronger . . . until you just have to resolve this conflict . . . it will feel so intolerable . . . [The therapist invites freedom in resolving the conflict:] And you will resolve it in a way that is *characteristic* and meaningful to you. [The therapist takes precaution:] After this has happened, I will say, "EVERYTHING IS OKAY." . . . Your tensions will immediately dissipate . . . You will feel comfortable . . . You will be able to share any inner knowledge about yourself that you may want to share . . . It will feel good. . . .

[The therapist takes further precautions:] I am going to ask the inner part of your mind to indicate by the usual finger signals whether it is acceptable for you to go through this stressful experience . . . Your "yes" finger came up . . . [The therapist reinforces the conflict:] Remember . . . when you have awakened yourself . . . you will experience this ever-increasing craving for the candy, along with your awareness that it belongs to someone else and is not part of your diet . . . This struggle will increase until it becomes intolerable . . . and you will resolve it in a way that is *characteristic* for you. Then, when I say, "EVERYTHING IS OKAY" . . . you will feel completely relieved and free to discuss everything comfortably.

Now take a deep breath . . . Let it out slowly . . . Let go and feel yourself relaxing as deeply as before . . . Soon I shall count from ONE TO FIVE . . . When I reach FIVE . . . give yourself your usual cue to become fully alert . . . ONE . . . TWO . . . THREE . . . FOUR . . . FIVE . . . Good . . . Wide awake and smiling. . . .

C: [The client stretches her arms, yawns, and rubs her eyes with the back of her hands.] That was good . . . I felt more relaxed than usual . . . The floating feeling was so strong . . . It would have been so easy to just drift off into sleep . . . I really felt that I was leaving the trance for sleep a couple of times.

T: Last week your log book showed that you used the "stomach-shrinking" imagery four times to reinforce the idea of space reduction. How is it working with your food volume?

C: I really think that this stomach image is helpful. It seems to me that I feel filled up with less food. [The client glances toward the end table.] It really feels very warm in here this afternoon. Do you mind if I take my sweater off? [She unbuttons her sweater and brings the reclining chair upright in order to remove the sweater more easily. As she pulls her left arm through, it sweeps across the end table at her left and knocks the two bags of candy and the microphone off the table. The cassette recorder is not touched.] Oh . . . Wow! That's clumsy. What a mess! [The client picks up the microphone with her left hand and places it on the table. Then she picks up the two plastic bags with the candy. Some of the candy has been dumped out in front of the chair. In her handling of the two bags, some additional chocolates fall out. The loose candies are all gathered up by her right hand, and when she has gathered up almost all that are visible, her right hand becomes clenched into a tight fist. Her left hand has replaced the partially filled bags alongside the microphone.]

T: I guess that little table is much too close to your left arm. I hope that the microphone wasn't damaged. Do you think that it is all right?

C: [The client's face is flushed, partly from the exertion of bending, but also showing distress signs. She is sitting straight up in the chair, breathing rapidly, obviously tense.] I think the mike is okay. [She speaks somewhat sharply for her:] I don't know why I feel so warm and uncomfortable. I really don't feel like myself. I was so relaxed when I came out of trance . . . but this stupid, clumsy accident made me feel awful. Such a dumb thing to do.

T: Your right fist is clenched so tightly the knuckles are almost white. Is there any reason for your right hand to be clenched so tightly?

C: It just feels good that way. I guess when I get this upset with myself I tend to get very upset and tense. I feel that it is better for all the tightness to go into one place like my right fist and stay there until I work it off than to spread out all over me.

T: Is there anything that you feel like telling me?

C: Only that I am so sorry that this stupid business interrupted my thoughts. I'm having difficulty remembering just what we were talking about.

T: EVERYTHING IS OKAY. EVERYTHING IS OKAY. You can relax your right fist, everything is okay. Look at what is in your hand.

C: [The client opens her hand and stares at the M & M's.] Oh no! How did these get there? [She sounds puzzled and surprised.] What a mess!

T: You can remember everything clearly and comfortably. It is all right to remember everything and to feel comfortable. The inner part of you will help you to understand. Let's play back the last twenty minutes of your tape recording.

The client and therapist listened to the playback on the recorder. This included the pretrance interaction, the trance suggestions for the posthypnotic conflict, and the interactions after the "accident." The therapist asked the client what would have happened to the chocolates in her right hand if the episode had been permitted to continue. The client was convinced that she would have found some way to transfer the candies to her mouth without becoming aware of the process. The client was tremendously impressed with the experience. She speculated aloud that perhaps she had spontaneously gone into trance when the posthypnotic suggestion began working in her. She said that she had not remembered the instructions given during the trance—that she had a spontaneous amnesia for these suggestions, and that this amnesia included everything to do with the chocolates. However, as soon as the therapist said "Everything is okay," she was immediately aware of everything. She wondered if something like this could be happening at home.

The postepisode discussion was continued until the client said that she was absolutely free of any compulsion about eating the candy. The client enlisted the help of her husband in checking up on her home eating, but could not discover any instances of "hidden eating" at home. However, her weight loss over the next ten weeks was completely compatible with expected loss on the high-protein diet. The client also became much more open about herself in the ensuing therapy sessions. There was a drop in self-devaluative comments, and she felt more confident that she would be able to maintain her new eating patterns.

The total duration of the experience was 20 minutes. Marked psychophysiological reactions were evident, and there was no doubt that the client experienced considerable discomfort. Nevertheless, the therapeutic gains warranted the added stress. It should be noted that the client was a well-functioning person, competent in many aspects of life. This gave the therapist assurance that the careful monitoring of the induced conflict could have beneficial effects.

The five chapters of Part II have presented a variety of hypnotherapeutic approaches in some detail. Principles for their use and descriptions of the procedures have been demonstrated with actual cases covering a wide range of stressful physical and emotional problems and situations. The chapters that follow in Part III are organized around separate clinical areas, the selection of which has been guided by four general considerations: The topic should (1) be important in the life functioning of many people; (2) include problems where psychotherapy is regarded as potentially useful; (3) have a reasonable literature to support the use of hypnosis; and (4) be one with which I myself have had at least some, and preferably considerable, direct clinical experience.

III

SPECIAL CLINICAL PROBLEMS

The Nature of Pain

PAIN AS SUBJECTIVE EXPERIENCE

"It hurts!" "It's painful!" These are basic statements indicating the existence of pain. Pain may also be communicated in body action, as in grimacing, for example. The only valid indicators of the presence of the pain *experience* are those communicated by the person himself or herself, whether vocally or nonvocally. When such communication is absent, there is no basis for inferring the presence of pain. This is true regardless of whether the source of sensory receptor stimulation is internal or external, and regardless of the quantitative or qualitative character of the stimulation. Thus, when the person's consciousness is altered so that there is no perception of pain at any level of consciousness, then there is no subjective experience of pain. The emphasis upon the subjective character of pain points to the potential for modification of the experience by psychological procedures, including hypnosis.

Health practitioners have made use of a wide spectrum of therapeutic interventions to provide relief from pain. These include (1) the administration of drugs (i.e., topical or systemic administration of analgesic, anesthetic, or psychotropic medications); (2) surgery (e.g., ablation of provocative sources, severing of peripheral nervous system transmittal elements, ablation of central nervous system perceptual components); (3) physical therapies (e.g., massage, heat, cold, competing pain, vibration, electrical stimulation); and (4) psychological procedures (e.g., prayer, exorcism, psychodynamic reorientation of the personality, altering pain behavior, relaxation, biofeedback, hypnosis). Each of these modalities has some relevance for the modification of the pain experience and is part of the repertoire of relief measures. The central interest of this volume, however, is the clinical utilization of hypnosis for the alteration of the pain experience.

Psychotherapeutic interventions to moderate the pain experience, including the use of hypnosis, can be considerably enhanced by an understanding of (1) contemporary theories about the psychophysiology of pain; (2) social–cultural–developmental determinants, including situational factors, that condition the individual's perception of pain; and (3) the significant clinical differences between crisis and chronic pain experiences. In this chapter, these topics are considered in turn.

PAIN THEORIES

The "specificity" and "gate-control" theories of pain are currently the most influential neuropsychological conceptions that attempt to account for diverse clinical and experimental observations about the reception of painful stimuli, the transmission of pain impulses, the perception of pain, and the modifiability of this perception. Although there are common elements in the two theories, the differences in their conception of neuropsychological function have significant implications for clinical practice.

Specificity Theory

The specificity concept postulates the presence of anatomically and functionally specialized cells in the peripheral and central nervous systems for the reception, transmission, and interpretation of pain impulses. Peripherally, there are free nerve endings in the skin adapted for the sensation of pain, as well as other sensory receptors. When stimuli impinging on the skin activate the perceptual sensory network, the pain impulses are transmitted to the spinal cord. The pain fibers connect, in the spinal cord, with a neuronal network that forwards the pain impulses cephalad (i.e., toward the head) via two main spinothalamic tracts: (1) the lateral spinothalamic tract, and (2) the ventral spinothalamic tract.

These pain impulses travel cephalad via different fibers at different speeds, forming coded patterns of discriminative information. Both tracts enter the thalamus and make connections with sensory neurons projecting to the somatosensory cortex. These pathways provide for the rapid transmission of pain sensations; they also carry identifying information about the locus, onset, duration, intensity, and other qualitative characteristics of the pain, as well as information about the nature of the provocative stimulus.

Some pain impulses proceeding cephalad via the spinothalamic tract connect with the brainstem reticular formation and the medial intralaminar thalamus, thus activating the limbic system (hypothalamus, amygdala). The pain impulses thus travel both to the somatosensory cortex to excite discriminative, identifying functions, and also to the limbic system to stimulate the affective–motivational centers of the central nervous system. Strong aversive behavioral actions, autonomic nervous system responses, and emotional reactions are evoked by the pain impulses. The affective–motivational–behavioral responses may be specific to the pain stimuli, but may also include other previously learned responses (defensive–aggressive) to threat. The affective–motivational responses to pain may persist even after the peripheral pain receptor activity has subsided.

The specificity theory (specific receptors–pathways–responses) is straightforward and has useful explanatory power for the perception of pain, especially in those situations where there has been a lesion or loss of one of the connecting neuronal elements with a consequent loss of pain sensations. But it is limited because there are some clinical pain phenomena with which specificity theory cannot deal. Examples include the persistence of pain in phantom-limb pain; the decrease or elimination of pain when vibratory or electrical stimulation is applied to the site of a previously pain-evoking lesion; and the strikingly low levels of reported pain in situations where special, strong motivational factors may be operating. It has been observed that injured soldiers may make relatively few complaints about pain once they learn that they are being evacuated from the dangerous combat area to rear-based hospitals. Survival euphoria seems to be able to seal off the pain impact of the tissue trauma.

Gate-Control Theory

The gate-control theory recognizes the functional importance of some specific pathways. The explanatory power of the theory, however, derives from the conception of the nervous system as able to influence the cephalad flow of pain impulses from the peripheral sensory origins through *centrally* originating descending "feedback" fibers that can alter the transmission of pain impulses at both the spinal and supraspinal levels. These descending feedback fibers can either enhance or reduce the flow of pain impulses by regulating the "gate controls" to be either fully open, partially open, or completely closed to the peripherally originating pain impulses.

The gate-control system at the spinal cord level operates by having the small neurons of the substantia gelatinosa (SG cells) function as the gate that regulates the flow of information to the T cells. When SG cells are turned on, they inhibit the reception of signals by the T cells and thus reduce the flow of pain impulses to the brain. When the SG cells are turned off, the "gate" is open and the T cells are able to relay incoming nerve impulses upward.

The pain receptor network includes nonspecific large-diameter, heavily myelinated A-alpha fibers; small-diameter, thinly myelinated A-delta fibers; and nonmyelinated C fibers. The A-alpha fibers transmit impulses more rapidly than the A-delta and C fibers, and seem to connect with the somatosensory cortex more directly and with fewer internuncial connections than the small fibers. The sensory receptor system also has large beta fibers that are associated with touch, vibratory, thermal, and electrical sensations. Stimuli that evoke pain tend to activate both types of large fibers. The large fibers act to provide identifying, discriminating, and localizing pain information to the somatosensory cortex, as well as to activate descending fiber impulses that activate the SG cells, which then inhibit T cells and alter the transmission of pain impulses. Large fibers may also excite SG cells directly within the spinal cord.

The small-diameter fibers (A-delta and C) transmit pain impulses more slowly via pathways that connect to the brainstem reticular formation and to the limbic affective–motivational system. These small fibers can inhibit SG synaptic activity directly and thus can facilitate the transmission of pain impulses to the T cells. The impulses from these small fibers can also activate supraspinal descending fibers to further inhibit SG cells activity and open the gate control for the transmission of pain.

There are thus two competing pathways. When the SG cells are excited either by the large-diameter sensory fibers (A-alpha or beta) or by excitatory supraspinal descending fibers, there is an inhibition of the transmission of peripheral pain impulses to the T cells. The gate control is closed to the passage of pain information from the periphery into the central nervous system. On the other hand, when SG interconnecting neuron synaptic activity is inhibited, either by impulses from small-diameter sensory receptor fibers (A-delta and C fibers) or by inhibitory supraspinal descending fibers, the gate control is open. Then there is a full or enhanced flow of pain information from the peripheral receptors to the T cells and upward into the discriminative (somatosensory) and affective–motivational parts of the cortical pain perception apparatus.

Finally, the gate-control system can be influenced by central cortical processes that affect (1) the limbic forebrain (affective–motivational system), and/or (2) the somatosensory cortex (discriminative system). In both cases, these areas can modulate the messages transmitted to the supraspinal and spinal gate controls. Positive emotions, such as joy, pleasure, and excitement, can cause the limbic forebrain to stimulate those descending fibers that contribute to the excitation of SG neuron activity and inhibit reception of pain impulses by the T cells. In contrast, negative emotional arousal associated with anxiety, fear, and depression may activate those descending fibers that inhibit SG cell synaptic activity. The consequence is an increased passage of pain impulses to the T cells and into the central nervous system. A change in somatosensory cortical identification of the painful stimulus (e.g., the shift in a pregnant woman's cognitive perception of incoming stimuli from "labor pains" to "muscle contractions") may alter somatosensory feedback to the gate-control system by decreasing the reception of pain impulses by the T cells.

There still remains the important scientific task of clearly establishing the existence of an anatomical–physiological basis for the gate-control mechanism. Until such time, the gate-control theory continues to offer a useful model or metaphor for a rational approach to the understanding of how various kinds of psychological interventions can alter the perception of pain. It also provides a conceptual framework for understanding how memory, learning, and expectation can affect the individual's appreciation of pain, as well as his or her response to the experience of pain. Gate-control theory also provides a rationale for such clinical phenomena as the decrease or total cessation of pain accompanying the local application of vibration, massage, heat, and/or electrical stimulation. The consequent large-fiber activation (both A-alpha and beta) would produce excitation of SG cell activity and inhibition of transmission of pain impulses into the central nervous system.

CULTURAL AND SOCIAL CONTEXTS OF PAIN PERCEPTION

The therapeutic amelioration of a client's pain depends upon more than an understanding of the facts and theories of neuropsychology and physiology. A very different set of factors also needs to be included in considering the nature of the pain experience. This domain is conveyed by the cultural, environmental, social, and interpersonal determinants of the pain experience. Pain is not only a personal perception; the social communication of that perception is actually part of the pain experience. How others respond to the signals indicating suffering greatly affects the further perception of pain, the behavioral expressions of pain, and the total experience of pain.

Traditions about the many aspects of pain differ among cultures, among social classes within the same culture, and among different families within the same class. Varying combinations of factors in a given culture (or class, or family) determine whether a particular behavioral expression of suffering in response to a given level of stress is rewarded (receives sympathetic acknowledgment and personal nurturance), punished (receives ridicule, rejection, or other negative response), or ignored (receives no acknowledgment or response). Thus, in some cases, emphatic behavioral communications evoked by relatively minor stress stimuli may be accepted as legitimate. This social interaction may encourage the interpretation of a much wider range of stress states as being really painful, as well as support a more profuse and extravagant social communication of the pain experience, than in cases where stoicism is upheld as a virtue.

A particular cultural context may ignore or punish expressions of pain where the provocative stimuli are regarded as minor or inconsequential. Sympathetic acknowledgment of the presence of pain may be reserved for a limited set of circumstances involving considerable stress. In this case "stoicism" does not necessarily mask the inner experience of pain or indicate a tolerance for pain without social communication, for the individual's *actual perception of pain* may have been correspondingly influenced by the cultural mores. Many studies have corroborated intercultural differences in the threshold at which pain is experienced, the tolerance levels for pain, and the social expressions of pain. It is possible that these differences had significant survival value for the particular group as it evolved in its geophysical, social ecology.

The therapist who would provide pain relief in a pluralistic society where various patterns of pain acculturation exist needs to remain sensitive to the possibility that a particular social–behavioral communication of pain may represent quite different levels of ongoing neuropsychophysiological activity and stress. The cultural influence upon the perception and communication of pain again emphasizes the importance of understanding pain as a subjective experience. The focus upon the learned aspects of the pain experience not only is important for the understanding of pain in the sufferer, but also offers change potential for the pain therapist. The social–cultural emphasis, however, does not set aside the awareness that there may be considerable individual variations on the basis of nervous system function and constitution (e.g., density of small-fiber sensory distribution).

CRISIS AND CHRONIC PAIN EXPERIENCES

The experience of pain involves several time considerations that are important in the planning of psychotherapeutic interventions: the time available for the anticipation of pain; the duration and frequency of the pain event; and the time that has elapsed between the previous episode(s) and the current (or anticipated) one.

The Crisis Pain Situation

The crisis type of pain experience is typified by acute and often rapid onset, limited time duration, nonrecurrence, and frequently a lack of similar experiences in the past. The pain may be of moderate to severe intensity. Not infrequently, there are life-threatening components associated with the cause of the pain. Surgery and accidents (external and internal) are the two most frequent kinds of crisis pain experiences.

In most cases, the crisis pain experience is therapeutically managed by the use of chemical intoxicants (analgesics, anesthetics, psychotropics) that affect stimulus reception, neuronal transmission, or the conscious perception of the pain. The combination of relatively safe, controllable chemical agents with effective biological life support systems has made the choice of such agents primary for crisis situations.

It should be stressed, however, that psychotherapeutic contributions to the management of pain in the crisis situation are not excluded by this "first-choice" use of chemical intoxicants. Considerable evidence exists to support the generalization that effective psychological preparation and support of the person through a surgical experience can result in (1) decreased use of intoxicant chemicals; (2) smoother, less complicated operative experience and postsurgery response; and (3) reduced pain experienced during convalescence.

Pre-operative visits by the surgeon and anesthetist may do much to moderate anxiety and tension, thus providing needed support to the person on the forthcoming journey through the unknown. Proper use of language offers both information and support, as indicated in the following examples:

"The medication you will get early in the morning will make you somewhat drowsy. It will help your body to utilize the anesthetic during surgery. I will be in the operating room with you. You will recognize my voice, even though I shall be wearing a mask over my nose and mouth . . . I shall talk to you throughout the surgery . . . Even if your conscious mind does not respond, your subconscious mind will be in touch."

Strong reassurance about successful negotiation of the operation can be inferred from a presentation such as the following:

"Some people expect a regular diet immediately after surgery because they have not eaten for such a long time. It will be necessary for you to have a light meal at first, but on the second day, you will most likely get to choose your own menu."

The focus upon diet conveys the confidence of the surgeon about safe passage far more than assurances such as this:

"You do not have to worry. I will be there to handle anything that may come up."

In the crisis pain situation, the person may be immediately required to cope with severe pain. The prompt use of a neurotoxic chemical agent may therefore be indicated. Yet even under such strenuous circumstances, emphatic therapeutic suggestions can have a highly potent impact. For example, suggestions of cooling and healing to persons who have just suffered severe burns not only can modify the perception of pain, but can also reduce the seepage of fluids into the injured tissues and facilitate healing. This example illustrates three goals of psychological intervention in crisis pain situations: namely, to increase the person's capacity to cope with high pain; to minimize the amount of chemical agents used, thus sparing the body the burden of additional intoxification; and to encourage tissue healing.

The Chronic Pain Situation

The chronic pain situation is characterized by the recurrence of stressful pain experiences over significant time periods. The intensity of perceived pain rarely continues at a fixed level but tends to fluctuate between episodes of marked exacerbation and intervals of some relief. However, even during periods of attenuated pain, the person retains an apprehensive expectation of the suffering that will come with the next surge of pain. The motivation to find relief from pain, to find lasting remediation, is therefore strong. The persistance of chronic pain seems gradually to bring about a shift of the person's life energies, concerns, and involvement to events associated with pain. There may be a concomitant decrease of involvement with work, family, recreation, and other life areas that previously claimed an important share of the person's activities. A narrowing of the scope of physical and psychological functioning may take place, with total disability as a dreaded end state, and loss of social and economic status as part of the preoccupation with pain.

The most frequent sources of chronic pain involve the musculo-skeletal system, with concomitant locomotor and postural disturbances. Examples are the arthritides, intervertebral disc problems, joint inflammations, tendonitis–bursitis–capsule problems, and low back stresses. The experienced pain is disruptive of motoric function and quite debilitating. The level of pain can be made more tolerable if the person becomes guarded in movement and action.

There is another distinctly more intense level of pain, however, that is so exhausting that it evokes heroic surgical and medical interventions. Examples are the pain associated with certain neuralgias (e.g., tic douloureux—trigeminal neuralgia); the ischemic pain of oxygen-starved muscles in spasm, resulting from some blood-flow-reducing arteriovascular disorders; and the pain of some osteolytic bone pathologies associated with metastasized cancer and periosteal infection. Leukotomies, rhizotomies, ganglionic destruction, and other types of direct nerve tissue ablation have been used to reduce the severity of such intractable pain conditions. The goal of pain reduction, however, is frequently not acheived or sustained, even with such radical interventions. It is significant that persons who have undergone leukotomy have consistently reported that the pain was still perceived, but that since it no longer produced fear, the experience became more tolerable. This abatement strongly suggests that the awareness component of pain and the emotionally stress-producing component, though related, are separate aspects of the perception of pain.

The persistence of pain over a period of time provides ample opportunity for many kinds of learning to occur that are related to the perception of pain. The responses of family and associates to the chronic pain sufferer, the social consequences of the pain experience, and the specific treatment procedures directed at modifying the pain experience all affect the perception of the pain and the meaning that the pain experience comes to have for the person. The pain may also serve the person in diverse ways—for example, in enabling him or her to control others or to avoid responsibility. In any case, the pain tends to become a medium for the expression of feelings of guilt, fear, shame, anger, worthlessness, despair, and depression. Self-destruction under conditions of severe pain sometimes presents itself as an attractive alternative to the continuous and ineffective efforts at coping with the pain. The chronic pain experience, for many individuals, thus leads to profound changes in behavioral patterns, self-evaluation, and outlook on life.

Whether the chronic pain experience is extremely debilitating or more tolerable, the sufferer may repeatedly seek help from a variety of health practitioners with differing types of approaches and skills in moderating pain: surgery, drugs, radiation, acupuncture, psychology. There is probably no other human experience that moves so many people to seek relief from designated social "healers" as the stressful, discomforting, fear-inducing experience of pain. It is to the hypnotherapeutic modification of pain that we now turn our attention.

Moderating the Pain Experience

The preceding chapter describes how the chronic pain sufferer may gradually acquire a life style characterized by preoccupation with the pain, loss of social status, diminished work involvement, and other separations from usual life activities. There may have been repeated experiences of helplessness and hopelessness, and the management of the pain may have been turned over to others. The chronic pain syndrome may be sustained by how others react to the pain and by secondary gains associated with the renunciation of self-determination and responsibility. Yet the toll in significant areas of personal and social losses may be too great, and the hope and desire for amelioration typically persist.

The use of hypnotherapeutic procedures for the control of pain is well served by the comanagement principle, a principle defining basic aspects of the relationship between therapist and client (see Chapter 1, pp. 8–10). Psychologically, the comanagement strategy is seen as therapeutically important for several reasons. First, it gives direct support to the ability of the client to function at some level to modify the pain experience—that is, to make a move away from the sense of helplessness toward self-directed coping behavior. The client also learns positive actions and exercises that can be practiced independently, outside the therapeutic session. Such homework reinforces client responsibility, contributes to the effectiveness of coping strategies, and helps the client to become reoriented to the nature of pain. Because of an increasing sense of personal control, the client gains confidence to risk re-entry into areas where previously he or she had been functional. Comanagement thus gives weight to the capacity of the client to make decisions, with support from the therapist, oriented toward relieving the pain. It supports the view that adequate coping is a process, not an all-or-none achievement.

Many clients find it helpful to have the hypnotherapy sessions tape-recorded. The tapes permit a more leisurely review of hypnosis procedures and recommended home exercises. In time, clients gain confidence that they can take over without the use of the recordings.

Occasionally, even with the availability of tapes, a client may ask to see the therapist for a "live" reinforcement of the therapy exercise, or an "update" that takes into account the changes that have occurred in the client's situation.

It is also important to allow for the possibility that psychotherapeutic support for the client with pain cannot always be scheduled in the form of traditional appointments. There may be need for frequent, short interactions with the therapist during the early learning phases of the pain-modification process; the therapist may have to come to the client's setting (e.g., the hospital bedside) during crisis periods to support the client's efforts. In any case, with the client taking an active role in the treatment process, there is much that can be done to moderate the stress aspect of the pain and to reorient the client toward a focus upon what can be done to expand the personal–social–vocational space, instead of remaining preoccupied with the constraints of the pain life.

INTRODUCING HYPNOSIS AND PAIN REDUCTION: EXAMPLE OF PROCEDURE

After an appropriate review with the client of the origin, course, and present state of the pain situation, the therapist initiates an educational orientation about pain and hypnosis along the following lines:

THERAPIST: You know very well how you have suffered with your pain and how hard you have tried to find relief. You may not realize that your pain is a combination of two things. One is the pain that comes from the hurt in your body, and the other is the pain that arises from the worry and fear this hurt has caused you. This emotional stress aggravates the body pain. Worry and fear put your body under additional tension. We know that this tension magnifies the pain you feel. When you become free of even some of this worry and fear, there is a drop in body tension, and you are started on the control of your pain. As you learn to put yourself into trance, your muscles loosen up; a relaxation of body and mind begins. Your whole being becomes calmer, and the fear becomes less. The pain that you experience becomes less, no longer as much aggravated by worry. The pain is already more tolerable.

More or less elaboration of these ideas is communicated to the client, depending on the comments and questions raised during this orientation period. The nature of pain and its control continues to be clarified in subsequent hypnotherapeutic sessions.

The covert hope or request by the client for complete abolition of pain is often accompanied by the therapist's own wish and pressure to help meet that goal. Yet the analysis of the experience of chronic pain in the preceding chapter makes it quite clear that persistent pain involves not only traumatized tissue and active sensory receptors, but also a traumatized individual whose life patterns have been significantly affected by the continuing discomfort.

The therapist can affirm the validity of the client's desire for a pain-free life without becoming bound by the criterion of absolute pain relief as the only acceptable therapeutic outcome. This can be conveyed in a presentation such as the following:

THERAPIST: It would be really wonderful if it were possible to abolish your pain completely. Someday, enough will be known about pain to make it possible for pain to be eliminated when the diagnosis is made as to why the pain was there in the first place. Today we know that pain can keep on even after it has served its purpose as an alarm, that many people have experiences that make the pain feel even worse than it has to, and that there can be lots of good help that will decrease the pain and make life more enjoyable even if some awareness of the pain remains. However, we can certainly hope that your pain will be reduced to the vanishing point in as short a time as possible for you.

The need for relief from pain provides a substantial motivational basis for the client to learn how to enter the trance state of consciousness. However, doubt about his or her competency in general may have become part of the client's chronic pain syndrome. The doubt engenders a critical attitude that keeps the person checking on the self to detect pain and determine whether anything is happening. This stance of a critical spectator works against lending oneself to the experience of shifting into the trance state. The therapist must be prepared to move gently, patiently, and persistently in the induction procedure, giving the client ongoing support until gradually he or she becomes more fully involved in and secure with entering hypnosis.

ASCERTAINING THE CLIENT'S READINESS FOR PAIN CONTROL: EXAMPLE OF PROCEDURE

How can the therapist determine whether the client with pain is ready to engage in learning self-management in the control of pain? How can clients who have experienced so much depletion of confidence be encouraged to risk effort in an uncertain venture? It is futile to ask; "Would you like to get some relief from your pain?" The client can only answer, "Of course! Why do you think I am here?" Perhaps a more accurate statement of the client's feelings might be: "Yes, but I have tried so many things and nothing has worked. It's up to you, Doctor, to do something that will give me relief." Complicating the matter may be the client's conflict over relinquishing the pain.

The client's review of his or her history will yield some notion of how ready the person is to venture forth. It is helpful, however, to seek further confirmation of the client's desire to proceed after the preliminary orientation to pain reduction has been presented. This can be done by introducing the concept of the inner part of the mind (see Chapter 2, pp. 29–30) to the client, and then by inviting further participation in this way: "Let us check first with the inner part of your mind to see whether it is okay for you to go into trance and experience becoming calmer and quieter within yourself."

The Chevreul pendulum technique or the finger-signaling method (see Chapter 2, pp. 29–31) is then demonstrated, and the question is asked: "Does the inner part of your mind want you to experience calmness and relief through trance?" A negative signal suggests the need to proceed cautiously and to work toward establishing greater security in the client–therapist relationship.

With ideomotor affirmation supporting conscious consent, the therapist may proceed with the induction of hypnosis. The client's reactions during the induction phase also serve as a useful indicator of the readiness to participate in the hypnotherapeutic comanagement of pain control.

In later sessions, when the ability to enter trance has been achieved, the use of future-time projection (see Chapter 6, pp. 90–94) can be employed to determine whether the client can envisage the pain problem as ever being overcome, thus providing additional evidence of client affirmation regarding pain control. As the client gains further understanding of the pain problem and skill in its control, the use of future-time projection can be repeated. The therapist can draw upon the client's ability with autohypnosis and ask the client to induce the trance state of consciousness. Then the client is encouraged to allow all knowledge of past events that gave rise to the pain to become available, as well as all knowledge of the present situation that sustains or alleviates the pain. The therapist suggests that specific images, words, or thoughts may come to mind, and that after a short while, a date will suddenly appear that will be related to the time when there is significant relief from the pain. The client is instructed to raise the index finger when this occurs and to communicate the date to the therapist. Then the therapist invites the client to go more profoundly into hypnotic trance so that the inner part of the mind can have access to even fuller knowledge about the self.

If the time selected for relief is very far in the future (sometimes to the point of indeterminacy), the client is expressing a multidetermined unreadiness to risk change (e.g., is too depressed to try, lacks belief in the self, fears the unknown). In that case, the client is given support by an interpretation such as the following:

THERAPIST: The inner part of your mind expresses uncertainty about relief from pain since the time is set so far in the future. This is understandable in the light of how much you have suffered and continue to suffer from this pain. Yet, during the hypnosis experiences you have had, your reactions clearly showed that there was a lowering of the pain discomfort during the trance. Somewhere within you, there remains some of that courage and confidence to control the pain. Let us assume an "as-if" attitude—that more confidence will develop as you try out new experiences and thus decrease your discomfort. After you have had repeated experiences of relief from pain, we will once again ask the inner part of your mind to predict a relief time.

Projecting a time for pain relief blends hope with the client's assessment of his or her capacity to achieve that reality. It may also be viewed as an index of the client's readiness to risk change—to move away from the existing chronic pain experiences and the personal-social behaviors associated with the life style of pain.

The extent to which the various procedures that have been learned are practiced outside the therapy session is a further indication of how committed the client is to controlling his or her pain. The point should not be neglected, however, that despite sincere efforts to become fully engaged in pain control, some individuals will need pharmaceutical support.

ROLE OF TRANCE INDUCTION AND ENHANCEMENT IN PAIN RELIEF

The very fact that muscle relaxation is part of the process of trance induction and enhancement means that, even during the early experiences with hypnosis, the client is beginning to learn the sine qua non of pain control. The therapist can maximize this learning by including various pain-related suggestions.

Example of Suggestions during Trance Induction

Images and concepts that have direct bearing on the client's particular type of pain can be introduced in the induction process. In the following brief example, tension release in the head, neck, and shoulder region, therapeutically indicated in the case of tension headaches, is focused on in the progressive-relaxation procedure:

THERAPIST: Tight muscles use up more energy and require more strain . . . Relaxed muscles mean a more relaxed body . . . The blood flow can move more readily to parts of the body where it is needed . . . The more the muscles of the scalp, the head, and the neck relax, the less pressure there is as a source of pain . . . the easier it is to dissipate a headache once it gets started, or to prevent it entirely . . . Focus on the muscles of your scalp, the frown muscles on your forehead, the squint muscles around your eyes . . . the biting muscles of your jaws . . . the determination muscles of your neck and shoulder region . . . Tighten all these muscles up slowly until you are fully aware of how much tension there is in each of them and how uptight you feel inside when these muscles are tight . . . Take a deep breath . . . blow out the air, relaxing yourself as you do . . . Let each of these head and neck muscles relax . . . the muscles let go . . . the uptightness lets go . . . the blood flow lets go . . . Feel the head, the scalp, the cheeks, the neck, and the shoulders becoming light and free as if a load were taken off them . . . the tightness going away. . . .

Example of Suggestions during Trance Enhancement

In deepening the trance state, the therapist can offer additional suggestions that will directly or indirectly support modifying the pain experience. These may bear upon hope, general positive affect, comfortable physical movement, and so forth. In the following example, several of these are highlighted in the bracketed comments. The demonstration involves deepening the trance through the use of number progression. It should be noted parenthetically that the extent of the count can vary and proceed in either direction, although it is advised that the particular direction chosen for trance deepening be consistently used by the therapist.

THERAPIST: [The therapist encourages positive affect:] Enjoy your relaxed state fully. In just a short while, I shall begin a slow count from TEN to ONE. In whatever manner is comfortable and meaningful to you, let a feeling start to grow in you as if you were floating, floating securely, comfortably, gently, freely, quietly. As you float along, let yourself imagine that you see markers carrying numbers from TEN to ONE moving by. They will seem to come by as I call them out to you. As you pass each marker with a number on it, take a deep breath . . . hold it for a moment . . . then slowly let the air out . . . Feel the air move out through your nose and mouth . . . You can almost feel the tension flowing out on top of the warm breath . . . and your chest, your lungs, and your whole body feel less tense . . . As the markers move by, the floating feeling becomes more and more complete. There is a lightness about all parts of your body . . . [The therapist suggests freer movement, hope, and personal expansion:] You may feel yourself so much freer to move, and your floating seems more open and free . . . Some have described this feeling as an opening up of the personal world, of hope growing, of a desire to reach out into the world again . . . Let your particular feeling of being free grow and as it grows, the tension goes down . . . Feel yourself lighter in body and mind . . . floating along the way you want to . . . able to control your own movement.

TEN. Take a deep breath . . . hold it . . . Imagine the number TEN marker coming by . . . See it as the first signal toward becoming less tense . . . Breathe gently . . . free of tension . . . floating along . . . Let the space around you expand . . . Let the feeling of lightness move into each part of your body . . . Feel the heaviness, the aches, and the fatigue begin to fade . . . The muscles let go as the stress goes out of them . . . Float along . . . Your body adjusts itself to where you are . . . feeling comfortable . . . relaxing . . . letting go . . . [The therapist suggests increased control:] Your own control seems to grow stronger with each moment that passes . . . Lightness . . . feeling free . . . [The therapist encourages positive affect:] It can be pleasant when you surround yourself with light, gentle colors or with images from your past that help you feel secure, safe, relaxed, free. . . .

NINE. Take a deep, slow breath . . . hold it in. Watch for the marker with the number NINE, another step in becoming more relaxed . . . Let the air out very gently . . . Let the feeling of lightness continue to spread to involve more and more of your body . . . Let the tension and heaviness continue to fade away with each breath that you take . . . As the tension moves out it leaves more room for calmness to spread . . . quietness . . . peacefulness . . . You may feel it more fully at first in some parts of your body than in others . . . It can be so interesting to see which parts of ourselves are filled by this light, quiet, calm state and which parts seem to take longer to make the shift . . . which part will next feel that calm, floating feeling replacing the heavy, aching, fatigued feeling . . . Your mind may begin to feel so much calmer and relaxed that it does not concern itself with which area will be next . . . What will be will be . . . Your mind feels the lightness within itself . . . Your thoughts become less heavy . . . floating . . . [The therapist suggests alleviation of fear:] Even the fears are lifting . . . If there is heaviness that still remains in some parts of your body, the heaviness may begin to take on a color or a shape that then becomes light and clear and glowing. . . .

EIGHT. Take a deep, slow breath . . . hold it . . . See the number EIGHT . . . Go past the next step of feeling the relaxation spread through your body . . . Your head and neck muscles feel so much lighter as you let the breath flow out . . . Breathe away the heavy thoughts and feelings . . . Breathe in relaxing air . . . Let your head feel light and clear . . . light and free . . . calm . . . [The therapist again introduces hope:] Open to new hopes . . . As the air moves in . . . your heartbeat will soon reach a steady rate that fits with the lightness . . . with decreased strain and ache . . . Feel the lightness and gentle restfulness flow in . . . floating . . . feeling freer . . . less burdened. . . . [The count will continue to ONE, approaching that point slowly or more rapidly according to the responsivity of the person.]

When the target point is reached, it is quite appropriate to introduce training for self-hypnosis. While in trance, the client is first asked whether he or she would like to achieve the same or even a more profound degree of quietness, calmness, and floating freeness through self-hypnosis. It is pointed out that "this skill can be of the highest value to you as you increase your ability to manage your pain experience." The finger-signaling procedure is used to affirm the verbal approval. Then the therapist may proceed with the autohypnosis training for relaxation and tension reduction.

EXPLORING NEGATIVE EMOTIONS: EXAMPLES OF PROCEDURES

The psychotherapeutic modification of pain views the affective component of pain perception as including much more than the immediate negative emotional stress associated with the current pain. Negative emotional arousal, whatever its source, is seen as contributing to the pain experience. The types of negative emotions that can serve to exacerbate pain are legion: Anxiety, anger, resentment, hostility, fear, worry, frustration, guilt, and shame are but examples. These feelings tend to develop defensive postures and muscle tension, which in turn contribute to the stressful feelings and the physical pain, and become part of a circular, self-sustaining system. Positive emotional states, on the other hand, tend to mitigate the stress level and to diminish the discomfort of the pain, again without distinction as to the source of the positive feeling state. Therefore, the examination of negative emotional experiences under hypnosis, and the resolution of their intensity, could serve to significantly alter the present pain experience.

A promising approach described by David Cheek in exploring and resolving negative emotions associated with one's pain history is to examine the *first memory of pain*.[1] The memory may be that of the client's pain or of someone else's pain. Questions to consider are: What gave that moment its special personal significance? Had anything been happening in the client's life just prior to the pain onset that was important? Was there anything besides the traumatic event

---

1. D. B. Cheek. Pain: Its Meaning and Treatment. In *Clinical Hypnotherapy* (pp. 142–152), by D. B. Cheek and L. M. LeCron. New York: Grune & Stratton, 1968.

that gave added meaning to the pain, that reinforced it (e.g., doctor's comments, guilt, personal loss)?

These questions can be probed while the client is in the hypnotic state of consciousness. The following might be said to a client who has become familiar with the concept of the subconscious part of the mind and with finger signaling:

THERAPIST: You already know about the inner part of your mind, the part that is not ordinarily available to you consciously . . . Now let the inner part of your mind get in touch with the first time in your life when pain, related in any way at all to the pain you are now experiencing, *first* became important to you . . . It might not have been your pain . . . It could have been the pain that someone else was suffering . . . When you are there, your 'yes' finger will move. As it lifts, those memories will come to a level where you can talk about them, if that is okay with you.

The psychotherapeutic goal is then to help the client deal with such negative affects and conflicts as might have been (or later became) associated with the "first moment of significant pain," so that their influence can become isolated from the present pain. When the total stress load decreases, pain itself becomes more tolerable.

After working through such a "first-moment" episode, it can be therapeutically productive to ask the client if anything earlier in his or her life might have contributed to the impact of this "first-moment" experience. Similarly, there can be exploration as to whether there were later moments that gave the experience of pain special meaning or aggravated its discomfort. In each of these instances, the client's decision-making responsibility is encouraged through the use of finger signals in determining whether there was such an episode that the inner part of the mind would now be willing to bring into consciousness. Whether these negative-affect memories are biographically accurate is not of critical importance. What does matter psychologically is that these memories, as part of the client's memory–imagery–fantasy complex, are actively linked with the present pain experience.

Negative emotional states are "tension generators" that contribute to the pain experience. In some cases, as in migraine, anger and hostility have been posited as primary agents in the buildup of an attack. It is important to explore sources of such emotional stress, alternative ways of viewing them, current tension-precipitating conditions, and possible action solutions. The hypnotherapeutic projective techniques described in Chapter 5 are especially suitable for this purpose—namely, the stage setting, the photograph album, and the hypnotic dream. It will be helpful to review these procedures at this time.

But what if a client is unwilling to explore sources of emotional stress? It may still be possible to engage the person in possible tension-releasing actions. An example is Milton Erickson's reported hypnotherapeutic treatment of a young woman who insisted that the hypnotic therapy be directed only to the relief of her migraine headaches.[2] After helping her to learn to go into trance, he gave her a set of instructions during the trance state, which she agreed to follow:

1. If a migraine headache or irritability should develop, she would immediately go to bed and sleep soundly for at least half an hour.
2. Following this half hour of sleep, she would spend at least an hour giving free rein, mentally, to aggressive fantasies: condemning, criticizing, arguing, and so forth. This was to be done initially in response to the therapist's instructions, but later because of her own satisfaction with this exercise.
3. After she had secured emotional satisfaction from these fantasized aggressions, she was to sleep soundly for another half hour and then awaken, feeling comfortable. She would remember only that she had gone to bed, fallen asleep, and awakened feeling comfortable.

The client carried out this procedure six times in the first three weeks, each time feeling comfortable upon awakening. Three months later, she reported having had only two headaches, both successfully managed with brief sleep. She attributed her freedom from migraine headaches to the hypnotherapy but showed no understanding of the therapeutic relief she derived from her aggressive fantasies while in trance. Fifteen years later she reported that she had about three headaches a year, readily terminated by a brief rest.

Sometimes, attempts on the part of the therapist and client to discover the precipitating conditions for a pain episode remain unsuc-

2. M. H. Erickson. Therapy of a Psychosomatic Headache. In *Advanced Techniques of Hypnosis and Therapy: Selected Papers of Milton H. Erickson, M. D.* (pp. 364–368), edited by J. Haley. New York: Grune & Stratton, 1967.

cessful. Support for what the client has been able to accomplish is then in order. The following example is that of a woman who had learned how to moderate her migraine, but who could not elicit imagery that related to possible provocations:

THERAPIST: You have made such good progress in being able to bring a migraine attack under control that it might be worth looking into how the whole thing gets started . . . Let's check with the inner part of your mind if it would be okay to look into how things get started and how to change them . . .Your right index finger said "yes" . . . Fine . . . Take a deep breath . . . let it out . . . Start counting backward from TEN to ONE to yourself . . . Relax more profoundly with each breath you take and each count backward . . . Drift back in time . . . and when you reach count ONE . . . some thought or image will come to your mind about how the migraine got started. . . .

CLIENT: Nothing . . . there doesn't seem to be any image or thought that comes into my head. . . .

T: [After two more unsuccessful attempts to elicit imagery] Sometimes nothing comes to mind. That can also happen . . . Just feel pleased that your inner mind alerted you to the warning signal of a potential episode . . . that you did not need to "tough it out" but responded with good migraine-dissolving actions that immediately quieted the blood vessels in your head and began your relaxation process . . . It just is working beautifully . . . If there had been some reason for your anger . . . you would have found a way for relaxing this feeling and then working it out of your system in a way that would not hurt you or those you care about . . . Your early-warning system is working well. . . .

Some psychotherapeutic approaches place stress on uncovering long-forgotten sources of frustration and anger; other approaches emphasize sources of stress in the here and now. In either case, the protected situation of hypnovivication encourages the exploration of alternative ways of perceiving and experiencing particular circumstances, whether historical or current, with the consequence that tension buildup becomes dissipated. Even laughter and joking can sometimes become a feasible alternative to anger and resentment. The importance of seeking appropriate action alternatives that lead to the discharge of negative feelings rather than to the inward storage of them is recognized by all therapies.

RELABELING AND CLARIFYING PAIN EXPERIENCES: EXAMPLE OF PROCEDURE

The name or label used to identify a potentially pain-evoking stimulus influences pain perception. A good illustration of this phenomenon comes from obstetrical practice. Many comanagement plans prepare pregnant women for a more comfortable childbirth with minimum use of fetus-embarrassing toxic analgesic or anesthetic agents. The training offers the concept of "labor *contractions*" instead of "labor *pains*" as a way to interpret the meaning of the signals from the pelvic area during the process of childbirth. The training exercises, each in its own way, teach the woman to induce trance in herself by focusing upon breathing patterns, movement of the arms, and muscle relaxation. The trance state is then used to intensify the mother's image of her growing child in her uterus, and then the image of the uterus contracting around the positioned child to facilitate movement down the birth canal. The process is pictured as a work-and-rest cycle, and the pregnant mother may be encouraged to watch the progress of her efforts in the mirror to give her access to visual awareness of what she is experiencing through her muscles and other sense organs, thus facilitating her involvement as observer–participant. The outcome of the training is generally a decreased use of toxic analgesics, thus reducing stress on the fetus and making it possible for the mother to experience and assist in the process of childbirth with reasonable comfort and to relate immediately to the newborn child.

Often it is important to clarify particular misconceptions that may have occurred under the stress of a painful event. An example of how readily misconceptions may arise, even when least expected, is the case of a patient who, upon hearing the physician say that the patient would have to live with the painful condition, translated the statement to mean, "If you are to live, you will have to have that pain." Clarification and relabeling go hand in hand.

A program for hypnotherapeutic moderation of pain perception has to begin where the client is in terms of his or her description of the experienced pain. Most persons carry some kind of mental image of their pain within themselves as part of their perception of pain. This image need not be well defined visually. The therapist may wish to help the client make this image accessible to therapeutic modification by encouraging the person, while in hypnotic trance, to describe it:

THERAPIST: Let yourself think of your pain as having some kind of image that expresses the suffering which you have been enduring . . . It will be an image that has meaning for you . . . It is often easier to deal with a difficult problem once we are able to define it more clearly . . . Let the image become clearer . . . Signal with your right index finger when you are ready to describe this image . . . Good. . . .

The image formulation encourages some degree of objectification of the pain. It also is a most useful source of symbols that enhance healing as alternatives to those that signal distress, and the therapist can reflect some of these alternatives back to the client as suggestions for reinterpreting the sensations associated with the perceptions of pain. Thus, the discomforting images of an infection, burn, or other injury can be transformed by an image of active healing, of seeing the skin as being rewoven and repaired by many busy cells. Terms such as "cooling," "soothing," and "calming" may be supplied as alternatives to "burning" and "itching."

One of the goals of moderating pain perception is to provide semantic alternatives to debilitating images. Whereas there is little room for positive imagery about pain that is labeled as "crushing," substituting the terms "squeezing" or "pressing" offers greater possibility of tissue recovery. The client is encouraged to select those healing images that have direct personal meaning and to intensify their vividness. An example of how this was done in one instance, using the complex imagery provided by a person with an ulcer, is given in Chapter 4 (pp. 67–71).

THE FLOW-CONTROL MODEL FOR PAIN CONTROL: EXAMPLE OF PINCHED HAND AND SWOLLEN KNEE

A great variety of images can be brought to bear to help the client gain control over his or her pain. The model of a flow system that can be regulated by the person is useful as a metaphor for teaching self-control of pain. The particular model that I have found readily translatable into therapeutic imagery for a wide range of age groups and educational backgrounds makes use of an electric circuit. In another of the demonstrations in Chapter 4, the metaphor of an electric circuit was used to teach the client how to shift the twitching of his left eye and cheek to a less conspicuous area (see pp. 64–66).

The client in the following demonstration was experiencing considerable pain upon bending his swollen knee, particularly while performing exercises prescribed by his physical therapist. Because of the pain history, I felt that it was important for the client, while in trance, to become more confident in his ability to control pain before the painful joint would be involved in the hypnotherapeutic experience. Using the imagery of an electric bulb, a light switch, and a heavy glove, the client was first helped to experience numbness in the back of his hand, and then was asked to pinch that hand as hard as he could. No pain was felt. The client was then instructed to push a needle through his skin. It was when still no pain was reported that the swollen knee was introduced into the pain-control imagery. As this excerpt begins, the client is already in trance; I am describing the metaphor that will shortly be applied to the hand:

THERAPIST: You know that all electric circuits are controlled by a switch that turns the lights on or off. Now there are also switches that can turn a light on gradually, bit by bit, until it is full of brightness . . . or can turn it down from full brightness, bit by bit, until it is almost out or even fully dark . . . In this way, you can change the amount of light to where it is most comfortable for your eyes . . . to fit what you need or can make use of at the moment . . . because sometimes a person may want to rest and yet have a little bit of light present for some reason . . . The nervous system can be seen as something like an electric circuit with just such a gradual switch controlling the flow of nervous energy into the pain receiving part of the brain . . . With your eyes closed . . . imagine that the skin and all the overlay tissues of your hand are becoming transparent . . . and you can see some colored wires that are connected to the skin . . . and these wires travel up the wrist . . . the forearm . . . the shoulder . . . the neck and into a central part of the brain where they connect to an electric light bulb . . . What color is the light?
CLIENT: Yellow.

T: Good . . . Turn that light on to full brightness and when it is all lit up, let me know by your right index finger's signal . . . [The client signals.] Okay . . . Now place that special regulator switch where it is easily moved . . . At your own pace . . . count to yourself while I count out loud . . . from ONE to THREE . . . turn that regulator switch so that the yellow electric light becomes only half as bright as it was at the beginning . . . and as you turn the light down . . . the flow of electricity to the back of the hand goes down . . . and with the turn down . . . the feeling in the back of the hand decreases . . . Not all feeling . . . just the pain and discomfort feelings . . . often feelings of pressure, warmth, and coolness remain even after the pain feelings are gone . . . It might feel as if a heavy glove were covering your hand . . . No matter how hard you or anyone else squeezes the skin or pushes a needle into it . . . it will feel as if this were going into the glove . . . aware of the pressure . . . but free of pain sensations . . . ONE . . . The switch is turning and soon the light becomes less bright . . . The skin is beginning to lose its sensitivity . . . TWO . . . The light is still dimmer . . . and the skin is feeling quieter . . . losing its sensitivity . . . feeling somewhat numb . . . THREE . . . The light is now only half bright . . . and the pain sensitivity is going down a lot . . . Squeeze the back of the hand with the glove on it . . . or whatever else is between the squeeze and the skin . . . Compare it with your other hand . . . You can feel the pressure . . . and the discomfort and pain are almost gone . . . [The therapist continues to count because some pain is evident:] Let's continue the count until SIX, at which time the light bulb will be dark, all out . . . and the pain sensation will be gone out of your hand . . . FOUR . . . going down . . . FIVE . . . almost dark and the sensation out of your hand . . . SIX . . . totally out, dark, the skin numb . . . Indicate with your right index finger when the electricity is shut off . . . Good! . . . Now squeeze the turned-off back of your hand hard . . . harder . . . It is interesting to be able to feel the pressure and yet feel no discomfort . . . Compare it with the other, turned-on hand. . . .

Now open your eyes . . . Take this needle . . . and push the needle through a fold of skin on the back of your hand . . . [Of course, the needle is sterilized.] That is excellent . . . Now withdraw the needle, close your eyes, and let the inner part of your mind register what you have just accomplished . . . You have turned off the pain feeling . . . kept it off . . . tested it out with the needle and found that you could do it . . . that you have the power to turn down the switch controlling the flow between your hand and the light . . . the pain receiver inside your head . . . What more is possible after you can do this? . . . Begin to count backward from SIX to ONE while I count out loud . . . With each count . . . turn on the flow of electricity so that the bulb becomes brighter . . . and the feeling in the back of your hand comes back to normal . . . SIX . . . The flow is beginning . . . FIVE . . . FOUR . . . THREE . . . When the light is half bright again, let your right index finger signal . . . [The client signals.] Good . . . TWO . . . almost fully lit . . . ONE . . . The lamp is fully lit and the back of your hand is with its full feeling . . . but you may notice something special . . . At the points where the needle went in and out, there may be a numb feeling that will continue for a while until the skin has healed the tiny puncture . . . then full sensation will be present . . . Test it out for yourself . . . Fine. . . .

[The therapist now elaborates the metaphor of the light switch to include not only pain control, but also imagery to facilitate the healing process of the swollen knee:] Now focus your attention on your left knee . . . See the same transparent process take place so that you can see the colored wires leading away from the swollen . . . hot . . . painful joint . . . Follow the wires as they proceed up the thigh . . . into the pelvis and then directly into the spinal cord . . . then follow the wires up the spinal cord . . . the back of the neck and into the head, where they connect up with a different light . . . and with a switch that controls the flow of pain and electricity to this light bulb . . . What is the color of this electric light bulb?

C: Red.

T: This bulb has a special quality . . . As you switch off the flow of electricity . . . another switch opens up that helps the blood flow more freely to the knee to cool it off and to bring more healing stuff to the knee while the pain is turned off . . . so that turning off the red light works in two ways . . . Now, let's begin the turning of the switch to cut down the electricity flow . . . and as the bulb becomes darker . . . the pain in the knee gets less. . . .

[The therapist elaborates the therapeutic imagery, and then continues:] Each time that you practice this exercise, you will become better at it . . . You will be able to turn off the pain for longer times . . . the healing will progress . . . and you will feel free to do the special movement exercises that support the healing process . . . If you should feel any discomfort during the exercises . . . perhaps the

light has switched on . . . Just take some time out to turn it off again
. . . The light will stay off longer and longer as the knee improves . . .
and turning off the pain helps the knee heal. . . .

There may be times when appropriate posthypnotic suggestions
about frequency of use of medications or other treatment needs are
also included in the presentation.

DIRECT HEALING IMAGERY: EXAMPLE OF MIGRAINE

Imagery that directly involves the healing process itself is helpful in
many cases of injury, illness, and pain. The use of guided imagery has
already been seen in Chapter 4, in the cases of a painful leg (pp. 63–
64), a skin rash (pp. 66–67), and an ulcer (pp. 67–71). It will be helpful
to review those examples. Presented below is an example from a case
of migraine, a not uncommon source of pain. The demonstration
illustrates the approach to pain management in which imagery involving the healing process itself is used.

Before the demonstration is presented, a few words on the
treatment of migraine in general are in order. The principal objective
in the control of migraine is to relieve the pain of the attack and to
diminish other psychophysiological stress reactions. The question is
not whether there should be dependence upon physical interventions
versus psychological interventions, but rather what is the most rational
combination of medication (e.g., ergotamine compounds, tranquilizing
agents, antianxiety drugs), physiotherapy, *and* psychotherapy. Prior to
planning a treatment regimen, there has to be a thorough life-history
review and medical examination to assess the possibilities of intra-
cranial pathology, systemic intoxications, or other physical states that
might give rise to the headaches. Not all severe headaches are part of
the "migraine syndrome."

During the early treatment phase, the therapist and client need to
explore all possible premonitory signals (sensory cues, auras, mood
cues, motor reactions) as well as situational factors that appear with
some consistency prior to a migraine. To help in this discovery, the
client is encouraged to keep a log for recording possible "triggers."

Numerous studies have suggested that a relationship exists between certain personality traits and a tendency toward migraine. The
personality profile is one of people who are ambitious, driven, perfec-

tionistic, domineering, righteous, and inflexible. It has been posited that these traits invite anxiety, frustration, anger, resentment, and hostility—emotions that lead to an overload of tension. It has also been posited that the typical precipitating event leading to a migraine is an incident evocative of such feelings, but because the individual cannot accept or deal with them adequately, the buildup of stress is discharged through a migraine attack. It needs to be stressed, however, that the concordance between the aforementioned personality traits and migraine is far from perfect. That is, there are people with migraine who do not manifest these traits, as well as people without migraine who do.

My hypnotherapeutic strategy is based upon four considerations about migraine headaches, and the belief that the client must become the principal manager of his or her own therapeutic regimen:

1. An urgent need is to promote cerebrovascular stabilization by diminishing the cycles of dilation and constriction of the cerebral blood vessels *as early as possible*, so that the pending migraine progression can be interrupted or at least abated.

2. The ability to become relaxed in body and mind must be developed. The method of progressive relaxation (see pp. 33–37) may be used, with an emphasis on relaxing the muscles of the head, face, neck, and shoulder region. Imagery directed toward reduction of psychological tension may be part of or may follow the muscle-relaxation process.

3. Moderating the fear of migraine is important. This is done by correcting the expectation of inevitable escalation in the course of migraine and providing coping alternatives (see pp. 153–154).

4. Where hostility, anger, and frustration are intrinsic to the migraine experience, the release of these feelings through appropriate action as an alternative to migraine discharge is an important goal of the psychotherapeutic process (see pp. 149–153).

The last three of these points have already been addressed in earlier portions of this volume and should be incorporated within the overall approach to the abatement of migraine. The problem of cerebrovascular stabilization is the main concern here.

One idea is that it is possible to reduce excess pressure on the cerebral arteries by having the person think or image the hands becoming warmer, once he or she has achieved a relative state of body relaxation. This notion initially stemmed from the biofeedback work carried out at the Menninger Foundation (Elmer Green and coworkers). Since then, research at the University of Kansas (David Holmes and coworkers[3]) has challenged the conviction that biofeedback involving temperature change is more effective than a no-treatment condition for treating migraine once the headache has started. The explanation suggested is that finger-temperature biofeedback does not alter blood flow to the extra cranial area so crucial for migraine. In the case of muscle-tension headaches, however, Holmes's research has shown that electromyogram (EMG) biofeedback is more effective than no treatment, but is *not* more effective than simple relaxation training.

In any case, because cerebrovascular disturbance is so characteristic of the pain experienced with a migraine, I have found it useful to gain the person's confidence in the possibility of pain relief by imaging the head becoming cooler and the hands becoming warmer *as soon as* there are premonitory indications of a pending migraine. In the hypnotherapy training experience, what is repeated in one way or another is that the resulting blood flow away from the head, coupled with body relaxation and quieting thoughts, eases the migraine. It should also be noted that the specific images during the training may be prompted by the therapist or induced by the person himself or herself. The latter is to be especially encouraged because of the particular significance and usefulness of self-generated images. Additional thoughts of quiet relaxation in general, and relaxation of the muscles of the head, neck, and shoulders in particular, are generally part and parcel of the hypnotherapeutic process. Sometimes it is helpful, as an exercise preliminary to the training, to have the person clap the hands or swing the arms in order actually to sense the warming surge of blood.

When the client has learned how to shift into trance consciousness and how to induce self-hypnosis, the blood-flow imagery may be introduced. Self-hypnosis capability is important since the client needs to practice at home and to become adept in using relaxation and imagery in preventing or assuaging the pain of a migraine episode.

The following demonstration is divided into two separate hypnotherapeutic sessions. The first session illustrates how the client may be introduced to ideas that will later be used in gaining control over a pending migraine attack. In this case, information is provided and

3. D. S. Holmes. Self-Control of Somatic Arousal: An Examination of the Effects of Meditation and Feedback. *American Behavioral Scientist*, 1985, Vol. 28, 486–496.

blood-flow change is experienced. During the second session, healing imagery is further developed and directly applied to the idea of cerebrovascular stabilization. Specific instructions as to how to forestall a migraine are then given as posthypnotic suggestions.

THERAPIST: [The therapist provides background information to the client in the waking state:] You know just what it feels like to have your head throb and pound during a headache attack. You should know that a most useful aid in dealing with migraine before it really gets started is to get the excess blood flow away from the head by imagining your hands becoming warmer, your head becoming cooler, and the muscles around your head loose and relaxed.

It is interesting that if someone puts his or her hands into hot water and applies cold packs to the forehead, the desired effect does not seem to occur. The use of imagination, of the inner thoughts, seems to set a process in motion that dissolves the migraine headache from within. With the body and mind relaxed during hypnosis, hand warming and other images become especially vivid and thus help in restoring proper blood flow into the cerebral arteries.

[The therapist seeks go-ahead from the client:] Do you think that the inner part of your mind is ready, at this time, to begin the process of helping you become free of migraine or of moderating the headache so that it is less disruptive of your life?

CLIENT: I wouldn't be here if I didn't want relief from these headaches.

T: I certainly respect that as being true on the level of conscious decision. However, it would be good to check the inner part of your mind with how the Chevreul pendulum responds. [The therapist proceeds with the ideomotor signaling:] That came very quickly . . . You inner mind also indicated that it is okay to go ahead.

[The therapist introduces prehypnotic exercises:] I would like to have you remind your nervous system and blood circulation of what it feels like to have the warm blood flow into your hands before you use your imagination in the trance state. Clap your hands together as vigorously as you can for three minutes . . . [The therapist could also use the arm-swing method mentioned above.] Begin. . . .

[Trance begins to be introduced:] As you applaud yourself for beginning to bring these migraine headaches under your control, close your eyes and focus your attention on the warm feelings in your fingers, your palms, your hands as the warm blood rushes into your hands . . . Feel your hands become warm with the clapping, how your fingers may be smarting a bit with their striking together, how your palms feel warm and engorged with blood, how even the back of your hand feels warm with the exercise . . . Good, now let your hands fall down to your sides and feel the blood flow down into your hands and maintain that warmth . . . Concentrate your awareness on that warmth in your hands . . . and as you do so become fully relaxed . . . relaxed and loose. [This client, familiar with the hypnosis process, readily follows through.] . . . Sense the warmth in your hands . . . [The therapist solicits imagery:] See what images come into your mind.

C: I can see a time when my hands were red and they felt just as hot as this time, maybe hotter . . . I had been playing in the snow for a long time . . . making snowballs . . . my mittens were soaked through and through but I didn't want to quit until my fingers began to feel numb and funny all over . . . Then I went inside the house and took off my mittens . . . My hands were very red and my palms were throbbing . . . My mother turned on the oven and had me hold my hands as close to the open oven as I could and then they began to feel very hot. . . .

T: That's very good . . . That's a strong recollection of when the blood really began flowing back into your hands . . . [The therapist suggests additional experiences:] There are two exercises that might further strengthen your awareness of what it feels like to have your hands experience a full flow of blood as they warm up . . . One exercise is to put your dominant hand into a basin of warm water. Then let the hot water continue to run into the basin, raising the water temperature . . . Concentrate on every sensation you can feel in your hand from the surrounding warmth . . . as your own hand warms up . . . becomes hot . . . Feel the warm feeling of your fingers, your palms, the back of your hands . . . Take your hand out when it becomes too hot for comfort. Repeat the exercise with the other hand . . . [The therapist suggests a home assignment:] It would be worthwhile to repeat this at least a couple of times before our next session together so that your body will be tuned in to what it means to have the blood flow to your hands and your hands become warm. . . .

[For the second exercise, the therapist again solicits supportive client memories:] The next exercise is to tune up your memory. Just as you had this strong memory come back about the snowballs, the numbing cold, then the redness, warmth, and throbbing with the warmup, there may be other strong memories of times when your hands really became warm . . . Continue with your eyes closed and put yourself in an even more relaxed state . . . Now let your memories stray back over any experiences when your hands felt really warm . . . If you want, you may even try out imaginary scenes in which you might experience hand warmth to see which ones are able to work for you . . . As your hands get warmer and warmer, stay with the experience and let your hands get as warm as possible. . . .

At the next therapeutic session, the client reports his or her experiences with the water-immersion exercise and describes the memories or fantasies that were useful in evoking hand warming. These provide the basis for further suggestions during hypnotic trance, as illustrated in the following excerpt:

THERAPIST: Why don't you do the hand-clapping exercise you did last time to get the blood flowing and your nervous system tuned in to warming up your hands? . . . When you reach a feeling of good warmth in your hands, close your eyes . . . Let your hands hang down by your sides . . . Feel the blood moving down strongly into your hands . . . [Trance induction proceeds:] Take a deep breath . . . Hold it . . . As you blow it out quietly and slowly, give yourself your cues to move over into a deep, relaxed, trance consciousness . . . Letting go . . . [Cerebrovascular suggestions are made:] As the body relaxes, the blood flow into the head region begins to slow down, the blood vessels begin to come back to normal size, and the blood flow to your hands increases as the blood vessels there open up . . . More and more into the trance state . . . the muscles letting go . . . [Supportive imagery is solicited:] Now let your favorite hand-warming image come into your mind to increase the flow of blood into your hands while your forehead begins to feel cooler and the blood vessels of the head continue to come back more and more to their normal size . . . Enjoy that hand-warming image or fantasy . . . whichever you choose . . . Let the inner part of your mind make all the necessary switches in the nervous system's wiring to increase the warming blood flow into your hands and the cooling of your forehead . . . [The client has previously had experience with the flow-control model.] And the blood vessels in your head and neck and shoulders are also becoming less full as the pressure decreases . . . The muscles in the head and neck begin to feel softer, quieter, calmer . . . They need less blood to function well as you become relaxed . . . [Dissociation from the body is suggested:] Feel yourself drifting quietly . . . drifting away from your body into a free, calm area . . . letting the body heal itself . . . Keep on enjoying your favorite hand-warming image while your whole body relaxes and your hand becomes warmer and warmer as it helps bring the blood vessels of your head back to a normal state. . . .

[Posthypnotic suggestions are offered:] At any time in the future, as soon as you get a warning signal, or find yourself in the early stages of a migraine . . . you can take any medication that you and your physician have found helpful in bringing relief. You will have a strong need to find a quiet place . . . and to shift over into the hypnotic trance . . . to begin your relaxation procedure and start the images going that are helping you feel so much better now . . . The blood flow will switch away from the blood vessels in the head, and the hands will become warm quickly and effectively . . . You will have no need to "tough it out" but will initiate the healing process as quickly as you can . . . The warmup exercise . . . the blood flow to the hands . . . the forehead cooling . . . your hands warming up . . . the tension-relieving exercises . . . drifting away from your body . . . drifting into restful sleep.

These basic instructions are emphasized as posthypnotic suggestions because they provide an alternative to being overwhelmed by the fear of the oncoming migraine. The client's memory of previous pain, nausea, other physical effects, and possible interpersonal difficulties is typically aroused by the first awareness of premonitory signs or initial sensations of a beginning attack. Fear and dread aggravate the problem and help to fulfill the prophecy of an inevitable progression toward the full-blown misery. Instead of surrendering to the previously experienced inevitables, the client is encouraged to react with an almost automatic mobilization of coping responses. Notice that not one, but a variety of actions are recommended at the first sign of a possible migraine: Proper medication, blood-flow imagery, cooling of the forehead, warming of the hands, body dissociation, and restful sleep are all included in the posthypnotic suggestions.

REACTIVATION OF PAIN-FREE MEMORIES: EXAMPLE OF INTENSIFYING AND RELIEVING PAIN

Another approach to pain control is based on the following premises: People typically retain memories of a pain-free period in their lives, with its concomitant physical and emotional feelings of well-being. A persistent pain experience, however, can submerge these memories. The psychotherapeutic premise is that clients who can recall these memories and experience a state of well-being, and then reactivate and intensify their chronic pain, can also learn to diminish that pain perception, even to the point of eliminating it. The imagery invoked during hypnotic trance is based on this premise. The therapeutic process can proceed along the following lines:

THERAPIST: You are familiar with your own signal for entering trance . . . So give yourself your signal to relax . . . to let yourself go all over . . . to feel yourself becoming light and free . . . Take the time you need to bring about a most comfortable feeling of calm and quietness within yourself . . . of the freeing up within yourself of muscle tension and inner tension . . . Raise your right index finger when you have reached that point . . . [The client does so shortly.] Fine. . . .

From what you have told me . . . you know that there was a time in your life when you felt well—physically, emotionally, and in every other way . . . when you knew what it meant to feel glad to be alive . . . when your body functioned easily and freely . . . [The therapist seeks permission to proceed:] Let's check with the inner part of your mind to see if it will be okay to go back to that time . . . to let the awareness of what it felt like to feel well return to you . . . Would the inner part of the mind use the finger signals in the way it has used them in the past? [The client lifts finger.] The "yes" finger went up slowly but definitely and remained up . . . Okay. . . .

[The therapist invites age retrogression in recalling wellness:] Drift yourself back through time to before the pain was part of your life . . . before the pain was in the picture . . . [Observer–participant dissociation is suggested:] Let part of you continue to remain with me in the here and now, while the other part of you goes back in time . . . Going back . . . going back . . . going back . . . When you are at that good time . . . Let me know by your right index finger . . . [The therapist encourages elaboration of the feeling of well-being:] Describe yourself . . . Tell how you feel in each part of your body . . . how it feels to feel good . . . Enjoy every moment of this feeling of well-being . . . Let every cell of the body restore the awareness of this capacity to feel well, which is part of that cell but which has been submerged by stress feelings . . . This feeling is still a part of you . . . Nourish it . . . bring in colors . . . sounds . . . or any other sensations you wish to strengthen that feeling . . . Let yourself feel very comfortable . . . Now count from ONE to FIVE slowly . . . and let all the psychological time take place that will revive these feelings of well-being strongly in your mind . . . Signal when you reach the count of FIVE . . . [Soon the client signals.]

[The therapist seeks permission for the pain experience:] Is the inner part of your mind ready to move up in time to the beginning of a typical pain episode? . . . [The client responds with the finger signal.] The "yes" finger says it is okay . . . [The therapist reassures the client:] No matter how intense the pain may become . . . you will be able to manage it . . . Observe what images are in your mind as the pain begins . . . tell me what you are thinking of . . . what you are feeling . . . [Pain intensification is suggested:] Let this pain become stronger and more intense . . . Feel it in all its typical ways . . . Let the part that is with me in the here and now describe it, while the part that is going through the pain episode feels it in all its usual intensity . . . If you wish, now make that even more stressful than the usual experience . . . This is a bad episode . . . [Pain moderation begins:] When you have the full awareness of pain . . . start the turnoff . . . [Pain is supplanted with well-being:] Let the inner well-being flow into your body and clear out the pain sensations . . . quietness, calmness, the muscles letting go . . . turning off the pain . . . leaving it in the past . . . the images of relief filling you. . . .

[Posthypnotic suggestions are offered:] The conscious part of your mind and the inner part of your mind will remember the importance of what has just taken place . . . Not only were you able to permit the pain to flow into your body in its very typical way, but you were also able to clear the body of this pain, to have relief replace it and the well-being feeling come back . . . [Homework is suggested:] This is an exercise that you will practice in between the pain episodes . . . Your skill at shutting off pain will increase . . . and then you will find yourself shutting off pain right in the early stages of your pain episodes . . . You will bring the pain into limits of feasibility that permit you to go on with your life . . . You can turn it off more and more as you gain confidence, and your life will expand once again. . . .

In the reactivation model illustrated above, three phases are evident: the reactivation of pain-free memories, the reactivation and intensification of the chronic pain, and then the quieting of the pain experience.

DISSOCIATION AND DIVERSIONARY IMAGERY

The psychological capacity for dissociation provides the client with a valuable strategy in the management of the perception of pain, as already seen in a few demonstrations. The imagery elicited in dissociation involves a "participating self" and an "observing self" as a means of moderating the perception of pain. The use of dissociation in hypnotherapy has been elaborated in Chapter 7 and illustrated there in the case of a woman who experienced excruciating pain while her burn dressings were being changed. The woman was able to remain in touch with her physical self as an intermittent observer of the events in her hospital room while accompanying her therapist on an imaginary walk in her garden. It would be well to review that case at this time (see pp. 113–117).

The participant part of the self is more readily perceived as *bound* to the physical pain situation than the observer part. In hypnotic trance, the observer aspect of self can be therapeutically encouraged to place greater psychological distance between itself and the physical self through concentrating awareness on its own activities as observer.

Psychological distancing from an ongoing painful event may also be facilitated without necessarily separating an observer part of the self from one's physical being. The therapist may help the client during trance to reactivate an experience of intense self-involvement, such as may occur during a theatre visit, sport event, or vacation. The fantasy trip serves to divert the person's attention from the immediate pain situation, thereby muting the perception of pain and in some cases even eliminating it for the time being.

RELIGIOUS IMAGERY: EXAMPLE OF
UNIVERSAL HEALING

Healers and clients with a religious orientation may draw upon the individual's religious beliefs as a way to marshal energy and imagery in support of well-being. The imagery may be stated in broad, general terms, such as the following:

THERAPIST: There is a deep universal healing spirit within you and in the world that you can draw upon for healing and for relief from pain . . . You must let yourself come closer to its essential meaning . . .

Forgiveness and love are parts of this universal healing spirit . . . that release the inner tensions . . . free your body and your spirit from pain . . . Let your thoughts focus upon your feelings of forgiveness and love . . . Forgiving yourself . . . forgiving others . . . releasing the stresses within yourself that generate tension through anger, hatred, resentment . . . And as the spirit of forgiveness grows within you . . . these tensions are released . . . opening up the healing life forces . . . permitting you to connect with the love of others and love of self . . . and love of God . . . As you open up to this healing love . . . the awareness of the pain becomes distant . . . moving further and further away . . . diminishing in importance and in consequence . . . as the healing love flows through you. . . .

Those who identify themselves with a particular religious group may invoke significant hypnotherapeutic images associated with their deep religious convictions. The client is encouraged to activate the religious imagery that will evoke the most intense religious involvement, including religious ecstasy, with a consequent distancing from the ongoing pain experience. The procedures not only emphasize relief from pain but also may provide considerable religious solace to the individual.

AMNESIA: EXAMPLE OF PROCEDURE

Amnesia for the suffering of pain experience can be helpful in two major respects. One goal is to decrease the level of anxiety in anticipation of the next episode of pain in the chronic pain pattern. The second major goal is to maximize the person's participation in ongoing life activities during the pain-low or pain-free periods. Even though, as the Hilgards have discovered,[4] there may continue to exist a "hidden observer" that notes and remembers the pain, the disruptive impact of the pain is reduced when the person does not consciously remember the pain episode. The person's attention and energy can then more easily be guided away from involvement with the chronic pain syndrome toward broader life pursuits.

The same general approach in teaching posthypnotic amnesia for

4. E. R. Hilgard and J. R. Hilgard. *Hypnosis in the Relief of Pain.* Los Altos, California: W. Kaufmann, 1975.

pain is used as in other cases. Usually the training progresses from forgetting simple functions (e.g., a word, a number, a sign) to more complex memory blocks. The training may take more than one session, depending on how rapidly amnesic skill is achieved. With preliminary training completed, the therapist may suggest amnesia for the experience of pain, as in the following example:

THERAPIST: [To client in trance:] The pain episode is gone . . . It is totally over . . . When the pain is finished . . . there is no pain . . . Only tiredness remains, and the fear that the memory of what happened remains . . . There was a lot of energy used up in handling the pain . . . and the body needs some time for the energy to build up . . . so you can go about your work and your plans as soon as possible . . . The resting helps the energy build up . . . The pain is gone . . . The fear serves no good purpose because there is no pain when the pain is over . . . And the fear remains only because there is a memory of what is past and over . . . Let what is past and over fade away. . . .

The pain is gone and there is no need to remember the pain . . . Instead, you can think of other things you want to do and can start to do . . . If ever the pain returns . . . you will deal with that pain as well as possible . . . With your energy restored . . . you will handle the future better . . . Let the fading continue . . . dissolving the memory of the episode . . . That whole experience is being wrapped up and stored far . . . far . . . away . . . [Feedback from the client is sought:] Let your finger come up when your mind is all cleared of the memory . . . like the wind disperses fog . . . and the sunshine comes through . . . [The client responds.] Very good . . . Take a deep breath . . . Hold it . . . let the air out slowly, and as you open your eyes . . . think of how well you feel . . . how the fog is all dispersed . . . far away . . . gone . . . gone . . . Wide awake. . . .

The effectiveness of the posthypnotic amnesia during the waking state immediately following should not be "tested." Rather, the forgetting should be allowed to consolidate while the therapist–client interaction focuses upon life-space-expanding activities. The client may need guidance through several sessions for the full effectiveness of posthypnotic amnesia to become manifest. Behavioral observation of the client's activity and comments by the client become the validating indices. This is not the kind of exercise the client can practice on his or her own.

TIME DISTORTION

Is it easier to tolerate an anguish that lasts five minutes and reaches an intensity of 10 on an imaginary Richter scale of personal suffering, than to tolerate one of 5 Richter units that lasts 30 minutes? We are quite a distance from a psychometric scale that can even approximate the answer. However, there are therapeutic circumstances where the negotiation of exchanges, such as intensity versus time, may substantially help the life functioning of the client. The concept of negotiating more favorable conditions seems to offer hope to some individuals who are unable to control certain stress situations, as in cases of phobias, obsessions, or physical pain.

The Ericksons described the use of both the expansion of subjective time and the condensation of subjective time in pain management.[5] One of their cases was a middle-aged, highly controlling woman who insisted upon relief from her migrainous headaches, which lasted from three hours to as long as three weeks, while reserving the right to experience these headaches when they suited her personal needs. In the course of several hypnotherapeutic sessions, she was able to accept the posthypnotic suggestion that, when a headache would appear at certain prescribed and convenient times, she would go to bed. The headache would seem to last several hours (subjective-time expansion) but actually would last only a couple of minutes. The woman carried out the instructions. Her need and right to experience pain were preserved, but the world time consumed by the pain episodes was drastically reduced. Also, the time and place in which the headaches occurred were more suitable than in the past.

In situations of painful medical or dental procedures, it may not be possible to reduce world time, but it may be possible to condense the subjective experience of time, so that time seems to pass rapidly (see Chapter 6, pp. 99–105).

5. M. H. Erickson and E. M. Erickson. Further Considerations of Time Distortion: Subjective Time Condensation as Distinct from Time Expansion. *American Journal of Clinical Hypnosis,* 1958, Vol. 1, No. 2, 83–88.

Becoming a Nonsmoker

PLEASURE AND THE SOCIAL–CULTURAL CONTEXT

The central problem of the modification of pleasure-producing habits is the very fact that the repetitive activities (the "habits") are pleasure-producing and reinforce their own continuance in terms of short-term consequences. The desire for change by the individual is motivated by a fear of future consequences that seem to make the short-term pleasures questionable, or by the cumulative negative consequences of the pleasurable habit that are beginning to counterbalance its positive effects.

Pleasure can be described as a positive cognitive–affective state of being, evoked by a particular activity. It creates a strong tendency for the individual to seek to maintain or reinstate this state. The state is often associated with sensations of arousal that are strong enough to be stimulating but not disruptive, with consummatory responses (physical or psychological) that decrease stress, or with thoughts and perceptions that support or enhance the individual's self-valuation (e.g., mastery experiences, goal achievements).

The events that give rise to this pleasurable state are strongly conditioned by the social–cultural learning that the individual has acquired. Each society designates many activities and events as acceptable for the elicitation of pleasure. These activities acquire their positive character through association with reward, approval, overt labeling as "pleasurable," and the myriad social supports that make pleasantness or pleasure an integral aspect of the occasions. Similarly, each society proscribes certain activities, designating them as sinful, harmful, damaging to the individual, and dangerous to society. This negative affect is implemented through punishment, social censure, creation of anxiety or guilt, and so forth. The activities then acquire a negative, unpleasant, distasteful affective quality and are avoided when the individual assimilates the aversive response for self-reinforcement.

There are cultures, for example, that negatively value and even forbid the use of tea, coffee, alcohol, tobacco, beef, pork, and so forth.

From earliest childhood, the individual learns that these substances are sinful, dangerous to the body, corruptive of the spirit, and threatening to the religious values of the person. Whatever sensory quality may be inherent in a substance, or whatever potential it might have for tension release, these values are readily perceived as part of the negative effect and experience with the substance. For habitual usage to occur, there must be considerable effort to overcome the "negative-affect" barrier and strong motivation to sustain usage in the face of this earlier conditioning. Those who do use such substances are pitied or scorned by those who are "enlightened" for their ignorance about the harm they are doing to their bodies and souls. In such societies, pleasure is associated with other activities or substances. The presence of a social context that supports abstinence from certain substances and reinforces the abstinence by aversive associations means that habitual usage of these substances is relatively infrequent.

The situation is very different, indeed, when these substances not only are designated as acceptable by the society, but are associated with celebration, social approval, and pleasure since early childhood, and are promoted by commercial interests as well. Moreover, if the culture emphasizes the "entitlement" of the individual to the maximum amount of happiness that can be garnered, then there is an additional strong social hedonistic context for indulgence in these particular substances or activities. Under these circumstances, when an individual considers giving up such a pleasurable habit, there is involved not only renunciation of the activity, but also renunciation of the social values and social context that encourages the use of these substances.

Every psychotherapeutic intervention that seeks to help an individual to modify a pleasurable habit must give due recognition to these two factors: the immediate pleasurable nature of the acitivity, and the social context that endorses and supports continuance of the activity.

GENERAL STRATEGIES FOR OVERCOMING PLEASURE-PRODUCING HABITS

Six broad strategies involving the direct modification of pleasure-producing habits are described below. Hypnosis is used to expedite and enhance their effectiveness by mobilizing motivation for change and rehearsing the strategies in the trance state of consciousness. The strategies reflect a variety of hypotheses about how a pleasurable habit orginated, is maintained, and can be overcome. It is desirable for the therapist to take advantage of the different strategies by combining them as needed in order to help the client achieve the goals that have been set. Each method has received support in the literature and I have had direct experience with all of them.

1. The strategy of future positive consequences focuses on the long-term rewards resulting from control of the harmful habit and the diminution of current negative effects as the frequency of indulgence decreases.
2. The strategy of negative accentuation emphasizes the negative consequences of the pleasurable habit and depreciates the pleasures by stressing their transitory nature.
3. The strategy of alternative means of gratification substitutes other tension-relieving activities for the tension reduction derived from the deleterious habit.
4. The strategy of conscious decision replaces the automatic occurrence of the habit by restoring a sense of responsible choice and control to the individual.
5. The strategy of environmental change alters the physical and social context that facilitates the recurrence of the pleasurable habit.
6. The strategy of self-reward invokes self-affirmation and other easily available rewards as reinforcers for each step taken toward reaching the goal.

The hypnotherapeutic use of each of these strategies is illustrated in this volume in the case of two noxious pleasure-producing habits: smoking (present chapter) and overeating (Chapter 12).

CIGARETTE SMOKING

The inhalation of heated air mixed with various suspended particulate matter (usually smoke from dried plants) is a worldwide practice, even in cultures with very limited contact with European societies. Smoking has a long history of association with ceremonial rituals, such as religious and social–political observances reserved for in-group members and for those who have arrived at the community criterion for maturity or special prominence.

During the two World Wars, a major factor in the dissemination of smoking among military personnel was their entitlement to cigarettes at drastically reduced prices. For many recruits at the training camps, the smoking of cigarettes became part of the initiation into manhood. During the first half of the 20th century, smoking was a male-dominated practice, but the use of cigarettes by women has escalated markedly in recent years. Pleasure, the achievement of "adult" status, the effort to emulate the "macho image," and peer-group enhancement have all contributed to the positive affective states associated with cigarette smoking.

Cigarettes have also come to serve many useful social functions. The offering of a cigarette initiates social contact between relative strangers and business contacts. The rituals of shared fire and smoke provide a basis for dialogue during exploratory phases of an interaction. There is a basis of action for hands and mouth during the social exchange. The smoking of cigarettes has become associated with a wide diversity of other pleasurable activities and sensations as well: There are eating ceremonials, where ending a meal with cigarette in hand signals relaxation to "help" digestion; toilet habits, where smoking provides the self-conditioning of anal sphincter relaxation; and work breaks, where smoking signifies time out from pressure.

There has obviously been great commercial profit in promoting increased cigarette use. Advertisers have not hesitated to appeal to the young, the insecure, and the vulnerable by associating smoking with sex appeal, social approval, achievement, and popularity. It is also probable that for some cigarette smokers, a self-induced hypnotic state associated with a focus upon moving smoke has contributed to feelings of relaxation and tension release.

Cigarette smoking is a pleasurable activity that exists across social class lines. The wealthy capitalist and the minimum-wage earner can smoke the same type of cigarette. The tremendous cost gap that differentiates social class in the grade of alcohol consumed is usually not present among different brands of cigarettes. It is easy for a diversity of social–economic–political systems to support the initiation of the young into cigarette smoking and the sustaining of that pleasurable habit.

The linking of cigarette smoking with future damaging consequences has a psychological unreality for most people, especially those who do not wish to change their pleasurable habit. The time dimension makes it easier for the cigarette smoker to take the stance of "unbeliever" and say; "There is no real proof that cigarettes cause damage. So many things can happen in 20 years. After all, correlation statistics do not say anything about cause-and-effect relationships." Lung cancer, emphysema, and cardiovascular disease are frightening prospects. Denial of these potential consequences relieves the smoker of fear, and may even emphasize the importance of immediate pleasures "just in case." Furthermore, antismoking activists can be seen as belonging to the same group of white, middle-class, egghead reformers who are always pursuing "do-gooder" causes (e.g., opposition to environmental pollution, protests against nuclear proliferation, promotion of racial equality). If the proponents of nonsmoking are devaluated, then obviously their arguments are of equally limited value.

THE HYPNOTHERAPY OF SMOKING

The decision to quit smoking, to become a nonsmoker, means a long psychological journey for the cigarette smoker living in a "smoker-affirming" society. There must be a progression away from straight pleasure, through ambivalence about cigarette smoking, until the individual is able to reach a state of readiness in which rejection of (or even aversion toward) cigarette smoking is finally achieved. The individual may express a desire or an intention to quit smoking long before the actual rejection stage is reached—often when he or she is only a short way into the ambivalence phase. The positive valence of smoking, however, is usually much stronger than the early negative disquiet about smoking. It is not surprising, therefore, that the initial intention to become a nonsmoker is easily overwhelmed by the strong countervalent social and pleasure-habit pressures to continue smoking.

Yet substantial numbers of individuals do become nonsmokers after years of cigarette smoking. What are some of the conditions that most probably sustain the decision to become a nonsmoker? The "quit-smoker" must have a capacity for envisioning the future-time period with some of the same feeling of reality that is invested in the present-time experience. Then it becomes possible for the presumed future-time consequences to be experienced as directly related to the present smoking of cigarettes. Furthermore, the "quit-smoker" must perceive the future as a desirable time in which to be alive, with a strong belief in the probability of being alive at that time. Then the identification of oneself as a nonsmoker carries with it many positive consequences that balance out the immediate pleasures of smoking, the discomfort of stopping, and the myriad of other adjustments required.

It is obvious that a cigarette smoker who is able to become a nonsmoker through his or her own actions does not need the help of a therapist. It is the individual whose own resources and efforts have been insufficient to achieve the nonsmoker status who comes to the therapist requesting help.

Exploring the Decision to Quit Smoking

When a client seeks hypnosis to transform the self into a nonsmoker, the plea is implicit: "Make this happen for me." My own therapeutic response is that I cannot transform the client into a nonsmoker, but that I will work fully and collaboratively with the client to help bring that change about, and that many persons have achieved the goal of becoming nonsmokers.

First, the therapist should review the client's smoking history, not only to gain a perspective of the ways in which cigarette smoking is part of the client's daily routines, but also to convey respect for the client's decision to become a nonsmoker. A detailed smoking history is taken covering the way in which the client was introduced to smoking, the pleasant associations with cigarettes, the negative feelings about smoking, previous attempts to quit smoking, and the social concomitants of the present decision to give up the habit.

The therapist then helps the client to prepare an inventory of all the pleasures associated with cigarette smoking. Each of the items is rated on a scale from 1 ("will not miss much") to 5 ("will miss very much"). A second inventory is prepared for specific gains that can be anticipated in becoming a nonsmoker. These items are also rated on a scale ranging from 1 ("minor importance") to 5 ("major importance"). The two lists are then discussed with the client as a method of further exploring the motivations for the change of self-identification from smoker to nonsmoker.

The therapist emphasizes that the decision to become a nonsmoker is a personal responsibility that no one can assume for the client, and that no one except the client can implement. The client is reminded that, on the face of it, it should be very simple to become a nonsmoker. All that has to be done is never again to take a cigarette, place it between the lips, light it, and inhale. No one else can smoke that cigarette for the client. Yet clearly, many people have considerable difficulty in sustaining that simple act of not smoking, even though there is nothing morally or characterologically amiss with them. The problem arises because smoking is pleasurable, strongly habit-forming, and highly supported by society (although recently antismoking pressures have become more widespread). Small wonder that the ambivalence about becoming a nonsmoker is considerable. Hypnotherapy can assist the individual to carry through the decision into action, but cannot either make the decision or carry out the action.

The use of the Chevreul pendulum or of finger signaling described in Chapter 2 (pp. 29–31) is presented to the client as the next step in exploring the decision to quit smoking. It is pointed out that the conscious, up-front reasons for quitting have been discussed, but that there is much in every person's decision-making process that draws upon the "inner mind," that part of the person that stores memories, knowledge, and feelings that are not always in conscious awareness. The "yes," "no," "I don't know," and "I do not choose to answer" movements of the pendulum or fingers permit this part of the client to communicate.

The therapist then presents the client with the list of smoking pleasures, and the question is asked regarding each of the pleasures: "Does the inner part of your mind consider that you are ready to give up _____?" In a similar way, the inventory of nonsmoker gains is examined with the question: "Does the inner part of your mind feel that _____ is important to you?" Finally, two crucial questions are posed: (1) "Is this decision truly your own?" (2) "Does the inner part of your mind believe that you are ready now to become a nonsmoker?"

The use of the Chevreul pendulum or finger signals not only gives the client further opportunity to express ambivalence as well as commitment; it also provides an indication of how ready the client is to make use of hypnosis. With sufficient indication of commitment and readiness, the hypnotherapy of smoking can proceed.

As noted earlier, the hypnotherapy of smoking draws upon a variety of strategies to help the client reach a successful outcome. The strategies may be combined as an integrated process or applied sequentially. For heuristic purposes, they are discussed separately here, although in some of the illustrations a number of strategies are intertwined. In all cases, exploring the client's desire and readiness to quit smoking is essential before proceeding further.

The Strategy of Future Positive Consequences

There are many ways in which anticipated benefits from achieving the nonsmoking state may be made vivid and reinforced through hypnotic imagery. The long-term rewards of health, appearance, self-regard, and financial gain are examples of benefits. While the client is in the trance state of consciousness, the suggestion of health and wellness may be intensified—for example, as the client draws in smoke-free air. The client's past experiences regarding one or another of the benefits listed in the inventory of nonsmokers gains may be evoked, and use can be made of future-time projection (see Chapter 6, pp. 90–94), in which the client elaborates the beneficial effects anticipated in his or her personal life. Guided imagery can also help the client envision the reduction and elimination of coughing, lung contamination, and other negative effects of smoking as the habit is overcome (see Chapter 4, pp. 67–71).

Health as an intrinsic value is emphasized in the treatment of Dr. Herbert Spiegel[1] as the foundation upon which realizing any future benefits of becoming a nonsmoker rests. The client is helped to concentrate intensely on three health axioms: (1) "Smoking is a poison for my body"; (2) "I cannot live without my body"; and (3) "I owe my body respect and protection." Elaborating and concentrating on these health axioms takes place in a single hypnotic encounter after the client's competency to enter hypnotic trance and make use of self-hypnosis has been established.

The therapist offers a highly persuasive set of suggstions as to why a full commitment should be made to these three axioms, but the decision is left to the client. Once that commitment is fully made, then the client has all the necessary power within himself or herself never to smoke another cigarette.

The next phase of the therapetic interaction focuses upon the

1. H. Spiegel. A Single-Treatment Method to Stop Smoking Using Ancillary Self-Hypnosis. *International Journal of Clinical and Experimental Hypnosis,* 1970, Vol. 18, 235–249.

importance of practicing an assigned exercise that, once mastered, takes but a short time. In the exercise, the client induces self-hypnosis and then repeats and reflects upon the three health axioms. The exercise is to be repeated ten times a day until the point is reached where the axioms become completely assimilated into the client's being, almost reflexively available to maintain the decision for health. Repeating the exercise ten times a day means that at no time is a recent practice period too far in the past to lose its effectiveness. Should the client suddenly find himself or herself reaching for a cigarette, the client can quickly mobilize the basic health axioms by giving the self a specific cue (e.g., stroking the cheek) to reactivate the message: "I owe my body respect and protection."

The client is enlisted as the comanager of therapy and given a rationale for each step in the treatment procedure. The emphasis upon the client's free choice places responsibility for becoming a nonsmoker upon the client, with strong assurances that commitment to the decision will bring about positive health consequences.

The Strategy of Negative Accentuation: Example of a Two- to Three-Pack Smoker

The strategy of negative accentuation recognizes that the habitual smoker accumulates many negative by-products from the smoking. Burn holes in clothing, foul-smelling ash trays heaped with crushed butts, hacking coughs at night, and thick phlegm that chokes the throat in the morning are but a few examples of the negative baggage that accompanies substantial cigarette smoking. The strategy focuses on actual negative experiences that are evoked by the imagery of these events during hypnotic trance. The client can draw up an inventory of negatives to be used for this purpose. Accentuating the negative serves as a counterbalance to the pleasurable affect associated with cigarette smoking.

In the following illustration, the client was a 42-year-old engineering executive who had smoked 40–60 cigarettes per day for at least the past ten years. He willingly accepted referral for treatment by his physician. There had been two previous therapeutic sessions:

THERAPIST: You listed two distressing experiences that were important to you in making your decision to become a nonsmoker: first, the heavy yellow crud that you have so much trouble in bringing up from your lungs in the morning; second, the ten to fifteen minutes of deep coughing and wheezing each night when you first hit the sack.

CLIENT: Right, both of them really worry me. They were part of the reason I saw my doctor.

T: There is no question about your getting pleasure out of smoking in the past and in the present. These two bad reactions can help you reach your goal of becoming a nonsmoker instead of just being things that have frightened you as threats to your health. I would like to ask the inner part of your mind if it would be okay for you to intensify the frightening feelings that each of these experiences arouses in you, so that these feelings are not just pushed out of mind as soon as the event is over, but that they remain up front in your memory. If you should reach for a cigarette, not only will you have a vivid recall of how you felt when these events happen, but you might even have the events begin right there and then.

C: I don't see how that would be any worse than what actually happens. I have had some terrible feelings about both of these experiences. [The client closes his eyes and relaxes and the right index finger, the "yes" finger, rises up.]

T: Good. Your inner mind seems strongly committed to nonsmoking . . . Give yourself the signal to go into trance . . . and drift ahead in time to tomorrow morning . . . You are in your bathroom, and you are ready to try raising the heavy phlegm froom your throat . . . Signal with your right index finger when you are ready for this . . . [The client's finger rises.]

T: Fill your thoughts with wondering how hard it will be to bring it up this time . . . Will it be slimy yellow or green? . . . Will there be some flecks of blood in it? . . . Feel yourself gagging as you struggle to bring it up . . . When you finally manage to bring it up . . . look at it . . . Feel disgust and anger at the cigarettes that have done this to you . . . at yourself for letting it happen . . . It will disappear when you are a nonsmoker . . . More smoking will make it heavier, slimier, harder to bring up . . . Tomorrow morning . . . when you clear your throat . . . flood your mind with these thoughts . . . More smoking . . . worse crud . . . No smoking . . . clear throat . . . Let the inner part of your mind consider this . . . Does it want to use these suggestions each morning for as long as you need support to become a nonsmoker? . . . [The client's right finger indicates "yes."]

Now move yourself ahead in time until night . . . You are just stretching out on the bed when the first coughing attack starts . . .

Feel how deeply the cough reaches down into your lungs . . . Feel the bed shake with each coughing spasm . . . It feels as if your belly button wants to pop out with all the straining to get the smoke poison out of your lungs . . . Feel yourself beginning to wonder how much more the lungs can take before the smoke poison is cleared out . . . No smoking . . . no poison . . . Tonight . . . if the coughing begins . . . focus on the coughing . . . how it feels . . . how hard your lungs are working to clear out the past residue of smoke poisoning. . . .

Each time you make a move for a cigarette . . . let each of these images flood into your mind . . . Feel the strain in your lungs . . . Then decide whether you want to smoke the cigarette . . . It remains your decision . . . The more unpleasant and vivid these images are . . . the easier it will be to become a nonsmoker . . . It is worth the effort . . . After you have signaled yourself to return to the here and now . . . the inner part of your mind will continue to rehearse these images and make them available to you immediately whenever you need them to sustain your decision to be a nonsmoker. . . .

Some hypnotherapeutic procedures involving negative accentuation do not limit themselves to actual life experiences of the client. The client may be encouraged to create highly aversive fantasies about cigarettes and smoking during the trance state, and then, with strong posthypnotic suggestions, to evoke these aversive fantasies and their concomitant psychosomatic stresses whenever there is a temptation to smoke. There are many other ways in which the negative-accentuation strategy can be adapted to a specific client's experience and competency. Some re-education programs stress leaving ash trays unemptied for long periods of time, adding water to cigarette butts that have been collected in a bowl and "sniffing" the concoction, or watching and silently condemning the bad habits of other cigarette smokers.

It is rare that the negative-accentuation strategy is used as the only or the central therapeutic strategy. Most commonly, it is one of several ongoing approaches.

The Strategy of Alternative Means of Gratification with Examples

For some individuals, the smoking of cigarettes acquires an instrumental capacity to gratify important needs, such as reducing experienced stress, moderating shyness and inadequacy, and identifying with maturity and sophistication. The pleasurable affect is often more a consequence of its association with the gratification of psychological needs than the physiological influence of the smoking itself. In any case, the desire to give up smoking because of its perceived bad effects on health may be counterbalanced by the many immediate gratifications associated with smoking. The strategy of alternative means of gratification proposes to cope with the forces that delay the decision not to smoke or deter the progress toward becoming a nonsmoker, through (1) identifying those personal needs being gratified by the smoking and (2) making available attractive nonhazardous alternative means for gratifying these needs.

Cigarette smokers frequently identify "helping me to feel relaxed" as an important consequence of smoking. The language of description varies considerably: "When that smoke comes out, it's just like blowing off stream," or "Taking time out for a smoke gets you away from the old grind." However it is expressed, the experienced stress reduction is the common theme.

Fortunately, hypnotherapeutic stress-reducing procedures can provide safe and healthful alternatives to the use of cigarettes. The learning of progressive muscle relaxation and the invocation of calming imagery during the state of hypnotic consciousness are examples. Some applications of these procedures are designed to meet the general need for lowering negative stress feelings and elevating a sense of well-being, whereas others are specifically directed to the "brief-break" experience. Basically, the procedures and exercises are the same as those also learned by the client who is anxious, phobic, or otherwise stressed, although there is a greater focus on content having to do with smoking and respiration in the case of a client who smokes.

EXAMPLE OF IMAGING CLEAN-AIR-FILLED LUNGS WHILE RELAXING

Let us first consider the use of progressive muscle relaxation (described in detail in Chapter 3) as applied to the would-be nonsmoker. In inducing trance with this procedure, a few suggestions that specifically refer to smoke and clean air are illustrated in the following example:

THERAPIST: Slowly draw your breath in . . . letting your chest expand fully . . . Hold that breath for the count of FIVE . . . Very slowly blow that air out . . . Feel it move out through your nose and mouth . . . Feel it carry out the smoke residue from your lungs . . . leaving your lungs just a bit cleaner with each nonsmoking breath you take . . . Blow it all the way out . . . pushing out the pollution particles . . . Fine . . . Now quickly draw in a full breath of clean air . . . Expand your chest fully . . . Feel the onrush of air through your mouth and nose . . . stirring up the innermost pouches of the lungs . . . Hold it for one moment . . . letting it out quickly . . . Let the rapid outflow clean your lungs . . . and your chest relaxes . . . your lungs rest . . . Feel yourself letting go . . . [The procedure continues with various muscle groups.]

EXAMPLE OF IMAGING A PEACEFUL SETTING WITH
CLEAN-AIR-FILLED LUNGS WHILE RELAXING

When the induction phase is completed, the progressive-relaxation process can be repeated with a strong emphasis upon healthful breathing in conjunction with calming imagery aroused by a particular setting. First, the client is encouraged to recall or imagine a setting conducive to a profound sense of peace, quiet, and freedom from all pressures, external or internal. The vividness of the imagery is enhanced by eliciting as much detail as possible from the client about himself or herself in the setting. The therapist assesses the degree of relaxation by observing the client's breathing pattern, body posture, and skin color. When the peaceful setting has been elicited and there is clear indication of relaxation, the therapist continues offering suggestions of relaxed, quiet calmness:

THERAPIST: Enjoy your sense of letting go . . . of feeling and being relaxed . . . on your vacation . . . with your friend . . . As we go through the muscle relaxation once again . . . it will be a relaxation on top of relaxation . . . drawing upon the peaceful vacation experience . . . with your friend . . . reaching into yourself as much as you let it . . . relaxing whatever inner stress you may have been going through . . . feeling the negative strains fading into the background . . . farther and farther away from you . . . and a flow of calmness . . . peacefulness . . . quiet lightness taking its place . . . more and more. . . .

Focus on your breathing . . . feel the clean air moving in through your nostrils . . . over your lips . . . down your throat . . . filling your lungs with freshness . . . Hold this air in the air sacs as it brings in the fresh oxygen . . . Now let your breath begin to move out slowly . . .

Follow the air as it leaves the air sacs, cleaning out the smoke residue
. . . flowing out through your throat . . . over your lips and through
your nostrils . . . With each breath that you take, say . . . in your own
words . . . "Feel the smoke-free air, the calmness and quietness flow
into my being.". . . And as you exhale . . . say to yourself in your own
words . . . "The strain and tightness is blowing out with each
breath.". . . Very good . . . Practice this for a few times now . . . In
time the inner part of your mind will take this over whenever you
relax yourself and begin to follow your breathing. . . .

Focus on your feet . . . Notice how relaxed they are . . . how
your toes, arches, heels rest inside your shoes . . . Gently tense your
feet . . . Permit the muscles to tighten while still feeling comfortable
. . . Let the muscles go . . . Become not only relaxed but calm and
quiet . . . saying to yourself as the muscles let go . . . "My foot
muscles are calm and quiet . . . free . . . light."

This exercise covers all the muscle groups, as in the earlier experience.

EXAMPLE OF IMAGING A "BRIEF BREAK" WITH
CLEAN-AIR-FILLED LUNGS WHILE RELAXING

The "brief-break" exercise is usually introduced after the client has
acquired some degree of skill in using self-hypnosis for stress reduction. It follows the general lines of this protocol:

THERAPIST: You mentioned that the first couple of drags on the
cigarette were really the main relaxing effect that you got from the
cigarette . . . The rest was just going on from habit . . . The main
effect was from the expanding of your chest with the deep inhaling
. . . and then the release of the muscle tension as you blew the smoke
out . . . You can have the same release of tension and yet protect your
heart and your lungs when you take your work break. . . .

See yourself in your work setting . . . signal with your finger
when you see yourself at work and it is getting to be time when you
are going to take a break . . . [The client signals.] Good . . . Now go
to a place where you can take a deep breath of fresh air without
inhaling smoke from your cigarette or anybody else's cigarette . . .
Take a very full, deep breath and count from ONE to FIVE while you
hold your breath . . . While you are counting . . . let the inner part of

your mind remember the full sense of quiet and well-being . . . Now let the air out slowly . . . counting from FIVE to ONE . . . and as the air flows out . . . feel the quietness and calmness . . . the hopefulness . . . flow in . . . knowing that the smoke-free air has cleaned out your lungs and also relaxed your mind and body . . . Repeat the deep inhalation . . . then exhalation . . . once or twice more as needed . . . feeling the release of tightness in your shoulder, chest, neck, and whatever else is tense . . . Bring the calmness and quietness back with you to the work . . . This is so much more than cigarettes were ever able to give you . . . And it gets better each time you practice it. . . .

EXAMPLE OF SUBSTITUTING A NONINTRUSIVE ACTIVITY TO RELIEVE SOCIAL STRAIN

The preceding examples illustrate how relaxation procedures can be substituted for smoking in helping the individual unwind and reduce stress. In some cases, there may also be a need to find an alternative means of relieving awkwardness in social situations. For the shy, socially uncertain individual, smoking a cigarette provides a structured and familiar set of activities that enables the person to divert his or her attention from the uncomfortable interaction by retreating to the details of the smoking routine. There is the package of cigarettes to be located, the cigarette to be extracted, the offer of the cigarette pack to the other person, the tapping of the cigarette on the package, lighting up, the disposal of the ash, and so forth. These are useful maneuvers for hands, mouth, and mind, and when a socially uncomfortable person makes the decision to become a nonsmoker, a void is created in the person's social coping mechanisms.

When a client has used smoking as "something to do" in dealing with social stress, hypnotherapy can help the client substitute an acceptable alternative activity—one that is readily accessible, pleasurable, and socially nonintrusive. The alternative activity is rehearsed in the trance state of consciousness as a way to abort the tension buildup, to be reassuring, and to provide time for the person to make use of other social skills that have been learned.

Before a substitute activity can be introduced hypnotherapeutically, the client must have experience with trance induction, must have learned how to use self-hypnosis, and should have been asked, either through the use of the Chevreul pendulum or by finger signaling, or both, whether the inner part of the mind is ready to accept a change in coping behavior patterns. With all of this as background, the client is asked to vividly recall a setting or episode where he or she experienced a strong sense of well-being and confidence. Should the client have difficulty in recalling such an experience, the therapist may ask the client to draw upon books, movies, TV, or theatre and to select some character with whom the client can empathize who had such an experience. The imagery is then intensified as much as possible in order to have the client experience it as clearly positive and supportive. In conjunction with the feeling of well-being and confidence, a substitute activity is introduced. An example of this is offered below; in this demonstration, turning a ring on one's finger is the substitute activity.

THERAPIST: Let this sense of comfort, of well-being, of confidence flow through your body like a pleasurable force . . . so real that you can feel it in your body . . . Some people feel it like a color . . . or a muscle sense . . . or an inner glow . . . Each person knows what it is, even though different words are used . . . It is more than an absence of strain or tension . . . It is a positive strength that is your own . . . that can grow as you learn to recognize it . . . that can help you to reduce big problems to manageable size . . . Signal with your right index finger as you feel that special strength in you . . . [The client signals.] Very good. . . .

[The therapist suggests the substitute activity:] As you enjoy that feeling of strength moving in you . . . gently let your thumb and index finger begin to turn the ring on your fourth finger . . . [The therapist identifies the substitute activity with wellness:] As you move it around, it seems to bind that feeling of well-being ever more strongly into your consciousness as well as into your subconscious self . . . making it part of you . . . belonging to you . . . yours to call on when you need it. . . .

[The therapist offers a posthypnotic suggestion concerning autohypnosis:] Should you feel stress building up . . . that thumb and index finger can begin to move the ring . . . and you will be able to put yourself in trance to draw on this sense of well-being, of confidence in yourself . . . Whatever is confronting you can be brought back into manageable size . . . to be dealt with . . . sometimes in part, if you are not ready to deal with all of it . . . And then you can either continue the trance or terminate it as you deal with the situation. . . .

[The therapist reassures and protects the client:] As you practice with this feeling . . . you will become increasingly secure in your capacity to cope realistically . . . You will be able to talk and act while in the trance situation . . . Even if you do not give yourself the signal to terminate your own trance . . . it will terminate when the need is fulfilled. . . .

[Confirmation is sought from the client:] Tell me how you will use this new skill . . . [The client presents some situation, step by step.] Very good . . . Now let yourself go very relaxed . . . and give yourself the signal to be in the here and now. . . .

The client is encouraged to practice the procedure and to use the ring-turning activity for self-induction of security feelings. The client now has a functional activity that can block the habitual reaction of discomfort and sometimes panic in social situations that in the past impelled him or her to reach for a cigarette. The functional activity provides the time that is necessary for mobilizing the self to engage in more appropriate coping behavior.

Another activity that may be recommended also makes use of a body resource: The thumb may be used to stroke the inner surfaces of each of the fingers of the same hand, beginning with the index finger and proceeding to the little finger. While in the trance state of consciousness, the client is given the suggestion that with each finger, feelings of reassurance and capacity to cope are enhanced. The finger stroking becomes the self-induction cue just as the ring turning does in the preceding example: It evokes a pleasant feeling; it provides a nonintrusive focus of attention that relieves social strain; it signals coping competency; and it gains time for the utilization of other learned social skills. These assists help to neutralize stress and support the client's decision to remain a nonsmoker.

Psychotherapy covering a variety of areas, as well as special training in acquiring specific social skills, may be necessary to help the client become socially more competent if the decision to give up smoking is to be sustained over the long term. As always, the therapist's theoretical orientation guides the character of the psychotherapeutic intervention, with hypnotherapy being used as a facilitative tool.

The Strategy of Conscious Decision:
Gaining Control over Automatic Smoking

The strategy of conscious decision seeks to restore control to the habitual cigarette smoker over each individual act of smoking a cigarette by having the client decide *consciously* to smoke that particular cigarette. A familiar experience of many cigarette smokers is the discovery that they are puffing away at a cigarette without any conscious awareness of having had a desire for a cigarette, or of having lit the cigarette. Habitual smokers readily recall incidents when they momentarily placed a cigarette in an ash tray, only to light up a second one, having forgotten about the one already lit. Only the comments of someone else made them aware of what they had done. In a sense, cigarette smoking becomes an autonomous action seemingly independent of decision making by such smokers. Some combinations of external cues and of inner perceptual stimuli below the level of conscious awareness apparently becomes sufficient to activate the pattern of cigarette smoking without the smoker's awareness of intention or action. When such autonomous behavior exists, either relatively or completely independent of decision factors, there is serious difficulty in maintaining the decision to become a nonsmoker.

The "cold-turkey" abolitionists who take the "all-or-none" path to becoming nonsmokers do not have to deal with this problem because they rid themselves of all cigarettes and associated smoking paraphernalia. The situation is very different, however, for the "gradualists" who, for a variety of reasons apparently valid for themselves, choose a program of progressive decrease in the number of cigarettes smoked over time until the nonsmoking goal is achieved. They continue to carry some cigarettes with them during the transition period, which may be short or quite protracted in time, and therefore remain exposed to the activation of autonomous habits that have had thousands of pleasurable reinforcements. The hypnotherapeutic strategy of conscious decision is typically part of a broader program of therapeutic support for the "gradualist" who has made the decision to become a nonsmoker.

The client in the following example had been helped to acquire various skills with the use of self-hypnosis, such as stress reduction, alternative means of gratification, and so on. However, it was still desirable for this client to develop specific mechanisms to deal with the "nonconscious" type of smoking behavior. The protocol used with this client is fairly typical of the suggestion pattern used for the conscious-decision strategy:

THERAPIST: The inner part of your mind indicated very clearly . . . with your finger movements . . . that you would very much want to have full control over each decision about whether or not you were going to smoke a given cigarette . . . that no one outside of yourself should make that decision for you . . . nor should anything uncontrolled within yourself start you smoking a cigarette without your right to decide for yourself . . . Very good. . . .

Give yourself the signal to become very fully relaxed . . . letting yourself go into a hypnotic trance in which there is a total concentration upon your right hand . . . Everything in you is focused upon that right hand . . . Your eyes are closed, but you can "see" that hand . . . feel it . . . watch it . . . and experience it as capable of acting on its own, as it has done many times in the past when it came to smoking a cigarette . . . Feel something beginning to happen . . . as if your hand is going to take off on its own . . . how fascinating . . . as it begins to feel lighter and lighter . . . The arm and hand follow a familiar pattern . . . being moved along by the old habits . . . as if there were a cigarette already in hand . . . Feel your arm and hand move upward toward your lips . . . coming closer and closer . . . Somewhere along this path . . . before this cigarette-carrying hand can reach your lips . . . a point that the inner part of your mind will help choose . . . the arm and the hand will become *locked into position* like a beautiful sculpture of marble . . . At this moment . . . whenever this arm is in that position with a cigarette . . . you will become fully conscious of the hand with the cigarette . . . and will have to make a decision as to whether or not you really want to smoke that particular cigarette . . . It is completely your own decision as to which choice you make . . . but as soon as you make a conscious choice . . . your arm and hand will become completely free to move . . . every bit of block removed. . . .

Sometimes before you make your decision about the particular cigarette and release your hand and arm from the block . . . you may want to quickly run through your health-axioms exercise [see pp. 178–179] and the deep-breathing exercise to reduce stress . . . but that is completely up to you . . . When the decision about smoking is made . . . that arm and hand will be completely free for you to move as you wish . . . Good. . . .

Let your arm rest on the chair again . . . and take yourself through the whole procedure on your own . . . Focus your total concentration on your right hand . . . [The client is given time to work through the entire process with a minimum of contribution from the therapist.]

Your inner mind will be on the alert to lock your arm until you have full conscious control over the arm . . . and the decision to smoke or not is a conscious decision . . . as long as you desire that control . . . This control will be fully operative when you are in the trance state and when you are in the nontrance state . . . Let yourself return to the here and now at your own pace . . . fully aware of all that has happened . . . available to you at all times as a further step towards becoming a nonsmoker. . . .

The client and therapist may repeat the training at later sessions if any episodes of nonconscious smoking occur. With the client's long history of pleasurable smoking, the complex problem of bringing about change in such well-practiced psychophysiological circuits is recognized. As the new conscious-decision strategy is practiced, it gains strength and contributes to the nonsmoking resolution.

It should be clear that there are many variations that are equally useful in the strategy of conscious decision. The client's particular smoking patterns, habits, imagery potential, and competency in hypnotic trance guide the collaborative planning of the given strategy. The particular imagery cited above has been consistently helpful for clients who set considerable store upon their own decision-making prerogatives. For those clients who have a preference for an "external authority," there can be an appropriate shift of emphasis; such clients can call upon an authority to block the unconscious, autonomous cigarette smoking.

The Strategy of Environmental Change

Cigarette smoking always occurs in a context of time, place, and circumstance. This context interacts with the pleasurable psychophysiological aspects of cigarette smoking to form a complex matrix of situations, signals, and reinforcers that facilitates both the initiation and the maintenance of smoking. Many associations with pleasurable gratification of the smoker's social, physical, and psychological needs are part of this matrix. The transformation of the individual from smoker to nonsmoker, if it is to persist through time, requires considerable modification of this environmental complex.

The strategy of environmental change for the support of the

decision to become a nonsmoker has two major components: First, the act of cigarette smoking is separated from as many of the typical settings as possible; second, new environmental settings are created (time, place, and circumstance) wherein there is a planned program for the smoking of *each* cigarette that the individual decides to smoke. Each cigarette that is smoked becomes a specific unit in gauging the client's progress toward the goal of nonsmoking. No longer are there any "autonomous" cigarettes—cigarettes that are smoked without notice, that are forgotten even before the cigarette has been discarded.

A baseline record of the client's usual smoking patterns is first required in order to provide a basis for planning specific changes in the pattern of smoking and in the environmental complex that supports the smoking. A record is kept of the time, place, and circumstance of each cigarette smoked; the degree of satisfaction derived; and other data that the client chooses to note. Usually a one- or two-week sampling is sufficient to document the major smoking patterns. The settings of frequent and infrequent smoking and of high and low satisfaction can be determined from the record. The client can add other settings of significance (e.g., examinations, or other stressful situations), even if they did not happen to occur during the particular self-observation period.

The therapeutic program introduces a variety of changes, such as replacing the client's preferred cigarette brand with one of low appeal and decreasing the availability of cigarettes. Thus, instead of purchasing a carton of cigarettes, the individual limits the purchase to a single pack; in addition, no more than a prescribed number of cigarettes are carried on the person (e.g., a four-hour allotment or six-hour allotment). The cigarettes are moved from their familiar storage places, preferably to a locked area that requires increased effort for access. The conditions for smoking are rearranged: Instead of smoking after meals or while watching TV, the client smokes on a rigid time schedule—every 90 minutes or every two hours, for example—and the client must leave the ongoing activity to go to the new smoking place. The cigarette need not be smoked at the given time, but then it is "gone forever." There is no saving a cigarette for another time. The activity is redefined as *smoking alone* in a special place reserved for smoking, with no other ongoing activity during that time.

The illustrations above are only a few ways in which the program of environmental change takes place. The smoking is separated from the habitual environmental context, and a new one for smoking is substituted.

Hypnotherapy contributes to the strategy of environmental change by providing the client with unusual rehearsal opportunities. Self-hypnosis or therapist-assisted hypnosis can be used to induce a relaxed state. Then the client selects a particular setting where there have been especially gratifying associations with the smoking of cigarettes and describes the total situation in detail to the therapist, especially any involvement with the smoking of cigarettes. At the moment when the client describes a movement toward the cigarette, the therapist intervenes and asks the client to "stop the action." The client is asked to see the setting as if suspended in time, and to consider the possible alternatives to smoking at that moment. Each of the alternatives that has a realistic connection with the situation is explored for relevance and acceptability to the client. For example, the client might consider changing the environment by leaving the smoking setting on some pretext in order to do a quick health-axioms exercise or a deep-breathing exercise; or the client might consider lighting up a cigarette for just one drag, immediately dousing the cigarette, smelling the wet end, and so forth. Each alternative is checked out through imagery and feeling tone, and one is chosen that the client feels is most useful for that setting. The therapist supports this choice, no matter what it may be. The client is also encouraged to explore ways in which the familiar context can be changed so that the pressures for smoking are reduced. The client may decide, for example, not to sit in a favored "smoking chair."

The approach of coping and restructuring is applied to each of the important contexts in which smoking has a high valence. As in so many other learning situations, success encourages further success. The client who has had several rehearsal experiences under hypnosis, and then finds that the nonsmoking alternative can be used successfully, experiences the exhilaration of achievement. The alternative provides the client with a method for changing the environmental setting and gaining control over smoking without disturbing his or her social relationships. This strengthens the client's readiness to explore further changes in environmental settings that support the cigarette smoking.

The "gradualist" client must be the central planner for investigating environmental changes. All contexts need not be changed simultaneously. Altering even one high-frequency context (e.g., smoking after eating) may be a significant achievement in reducing the total number of cigarettes smoked per day. The client is also reminded that the strategy of environmental change is only one of the various strategies being used in becoming a nonsmoker.

It is expected that the "gradualist" will experience difficult periods along the path to the nonsmoker goal. Some environmental contexts (e.g., cocktail parties) may be just too powerful for the time being for the client to feel strong enough to deal with. The client may then be encouraged to bypass such a social context until his or her coping capacity has increased. The therapist respects the client's judgment. The client is helped to recognize that the learning of alternate means of gratification and the positive consequences of becoming a nonsmoker build up with time, so that previously avoided situations become manageable after a while.

The Strategy of Self-Reward

The last strategy to be discussed here is the strategy of self-affirmation, of rewarding oneself for progress made along the road toward becoming a nonsmoker. It means that subgoals are set that can be reached, and when they are reached, the client does not disregard or invalidate the achievement but notes it with pleasure and satisfaction, marking it as an occasion for endorsing the self. The principal beneficiary of the shift from smoking status to nonsmoking status is the client, and it is the client's responsibility to acknowledge each achievement that advances his or her own well-being. The strategy encourages the client to recognize that the remaking of years of habitual behavior requires many successful efforts in the acquisition of new habits and patterns of response. The large goal must be subdivided into smaller units, some so small that they deal only with a short unit of time, so that achievement can occur on a daily basis.

The priniciple of frequent experiences with successful accomplishment in the early stages of a difficult undertaking is a sound basis for later establishing more difficult levels of aspiration. Being able to postpone the smoking of the day's first cigarette for one or two hours should be appreciated by the client and associated with a specific affirming reward. Later, a delay of half a day or longer may be required to merit the same level of affirmation. The reward should be readily available and of known positive worth to the client: A special TV show, a phonograph record, a mark on a chart of progress, a phone call to a friend, and a game of ball are a few examples. Self-reward is easily integrated into the keeping of a diary or some other record of one's progress toward becoming a nonsmoker. Achievement can be indicated by stars or special comments. To the outsider, these indications of self-reward and praise may seem childish but to the client who is dealing with problems of smoking, these achievements are noteworthy. The client should be encouraged to use a language of pleasure in rewarding the self (e.g., "That was really great—no smoking for the whole morning").

Hypnotherapy can be used to enhance the celebration of self for the achievement of even small gains. I support the client's use of self-induced trance at the end of the day prior to bedtime in order to consolidate the progress that has been made toward becoming a nonsmoker. The client selects a special place where there can be an undisturbed period of relaxation. The trance state is induced and there is a release of whatever muscle tensions is a residue of the day's stress.

The client then reviews the specific achievements of that day. There may have been only one, or there may have been many steps taken toward becoming a nonsmoker. The focus is upon what was accomplished—what *was* done, not upon what *should have been* done. The client is encouraged to affirm this progress verbally to himself or herself: "I am more of a nonsmoker today than I was yesterday. I have moved myself closer toward freedom from the need to smoke. This is good."

The self-affirmation is then followed by vivid imagery based upon the client's specific motivations for becoming a nonsmoker: for example, an image of lungs that are clean and free of pollution, or of a heart beating regularly with healthy circulation. The image may be a stylized anatomical image, or some symbolic image (e.g., jogging or dancing with ease) that embodies the client's health goals. In the final part of the self-affirmation, the client focuses upon an image of well-being and high self-regard. The entire exercise need not take more than a few minutes, although the client is free to decide the total length of time. It also becomes a restatement of the intent not to smoke, with an implied or explicit posthypnotic suggestion for the next day's activities: "As with alcoholism, I am a nonsmoker for only one day at a time for the rest of my life."

FURTHER CONSIDERATIONS IN
EFFECTIVE TREATMENT

Effective progress by the client toward the goal of becoming a nonsmoker sometimes brings about other problems. Probably the most frequently reported problem is that of weight gain. This may partly be due to a heightening of those senses that make eating more tasteful. Again and again clients report that they experience a return of taste and smell once the use of cigarettes has dropped below the level of 10–12 per day. It has been described as feeling as though a plastic film had been peeled away from the interior of the nose and from around the tongue and the inside of the mouth. There develops an awareness of scents, aromas, and tastes that has been gone for a long time. Foods begin to taste better, appetite is enhanced, and more food is eaten. Some clients report that the recurrent experience of "sour stomach" seems to become less frequent and less intense, and may even disappear. For others, the increase of food intake may relate to a need for oral gratification; it may serve as a "substitute" for the special oral needs that were met by the cigarette between the lips. Whatever the source for the increased food intake, the weight gain may become a barrier to progress toward nonsmoking goals.

Three ideas may be presented to the client as a basis for coping with this problem:

1. The weight gain can be temporary. The client will retain the improved sensations of taste and smell, because these are restorations of what had existed before cigarette smoking obliterated them. The renewed awareness of taste and smell will become reintegrated into the client's everyday living and will be accepted as how food should taste. With that, the overstimulation of appetite is likely to decrease, making it easier to maintain proper eating habits.

2. The health priority associated with nonsmoking should be sustained by the client and should take precedence over concern with weight gain until the nonsmoking behavior patterns are firmly established. Attention can then be focused upon weight management if weight is still a concern.

3. The confidence in self, the skills that have been learned, and the experience with control over one's decisions have all been strengthened during the nonsmoker treatment and will be readily available to the client in coping with establishing the desired weight level.

Management of constipation, control of rampant antismoking zealotism (e.g., carrying the crusade into the camps of the enemy), and feelings of depression are other problems that may arise in conjunction with the client's decision to shift from a habitual hedonistic behavior pattern to one where enlightened self-interest is the prime determinant. The problems have to be dealt with as part of the broad-ranging psychotherapeutic process, with hypnosis being used to facilitate the changes. These problems are not unique to smoking. They are part of the realities of change whenever a client decides to renounce short-term pleasures for the sake of achieving long-term health or other goals related to personal well-being.

Obesity: The Management of Overeating

PSYCHOSOCIAL ASPECTS OF FOOD

Food as Survival

Abundance of food has been part of the human experience for only a short time—probably less than one percent of the known existence of humans as a distinct species. Hunger, even famine, is still very much a part of reality, part of the everyday experience of substantial numbers of our contemporary world's peoples. The availability of food to our forebears depended upon their individual and collective knowledge and skill in foraging for edible vegetation, and in successful hunting and fishing. It was typical for humans to experience regular alternations between fast and feast. Much, much time was to pass in the course of human evolution before the secrets of food preservation—dehydration, smoking, salting—would become part of folk knowledge, so that food could be stored after immediate energy needs were satisfied.

In earlier times, only one food storage resource was available: namely, the capacity of the individual's own body to transform excess calories into stored adipose tissue. Survival was therefore dependent not only upon the capacity to obtain food, but also, it is reasonable to assume, upon the individual's capacity to readily assimilate small or large quantities of food, and to easily transform excess food intake into stored energy (fat). Eating regularly, three or more times a day, was not and has not been available to humankind for most of its evolutionary history. The evolutionary process undoubtedly favored the children of those women who more effectively stored food throughout their pregnancy. Because of the unreliability of the external food supply, these children would have a more assured food supply during the critical developmental period *in utero* and in the crucial early months of infancy.

Throughout most of humankind's existence, the physical demands involved in gathering food and protecting oneself against destructive forces left very little possibility for accumulating an excess of input energy over output demands. Thus, even slightly more efficient storers of food had a survival advantage in the long time span of this selective refining process. The wide geographic distribution of human beings—from the tropics to the Arctic Circle, from the seashores to the high mountain ranges—made special demands not only upon this capacity to store energy, but also upon where in the body this stored tissue (fat) would be most advantageous to survival under these varied conditions. Body proportions, muscle-to-fat ratios, and many other factors of body structure were influenced by these environmental factors.

Given this history of adaptation for survival within an economy of food scarcity, the human body was not well prepared for food abundance.

Food and the Celebration of Life

Eating to fullness, even to the point of maximum stomach capacity, was a practical necessity of life in a world of uncertain food supply and no storage facilities. The full stomach signaled a temporary respite from the all-too-familiar hunger sensations. The sense of physical well-being associated with food assimilation was accompanied by psychological relaxation related to the lowered urgency for food gathering. Such occasions were periods, intermittent, infrequent, and brief, when there was enough "surplus energy" for the elaboration of social communication; at these times, customs, rituals, beliefs, and ceremonials evolved to indicate grateful acknowledgment for the food, the sustainer of life, and to express the hope and need for early and frequent recurrences of the same benificence. The celebration of the successful hunt was also a celebration of the extension of existence made possible by the renewed supply of food.

The human capacity for social cohesion and communication had magnified the individual's food-gathering capacity and survival. The evolution of significant social symbolism with each aspect of food further emphasized the importance of collective action in the obtaining and utilization of food. The hunting–migratory pattern of human existence covered a far larger proportion of the history of humankind than the relatively recent agricultural mode, and the social symbols dealing with food have had a long evolution in becoming embedded in so many aspects of human life.

Cultivation of the soil and the domestication of animals for food profoundly altered the hunting–migratory life style and also provided the possibility of a more stable and expanded food supply. Even with only a pointed stick and human muscle power to provide the energy for turning the soil, the planting of seeds immeasurably extended control over the environment. The evolution of the food storage potential (through grains and food animals) meant that the extreme fluctuations of fast and feast could be moderated, that all available food did not have to be consumed before it spoiled, and that more modest amounts could be eaten each day.

The important social symbolizations associated with the many aspects of food in the hunting society were incorporated into the agricultural life pattern: Instead of the successful hunt, the planting and harvesting of food became important occasions. As the storage of food outside the body became an increasing reality, other events became marked by "food celebrations." Birth, maturation, marriage, and death become occasions for important rituals and ceremonials. In the life of the community, leadership changes, community undertakings, and other designated events besides planting and harvesting became occasions for special food ceremonials, with elaborate specifications of kinds of food, ways of eating, choice of celebrants, and so forth.

Thus, far beyond its basic nutritional necessity, food has been an important part of the celebration of significant life events throughout human existence. A close association among food, pleasure, well-being, and achievement is assured in each individual's life through the impact of language, social customs, and personal developmental experiences.

Food as a Source of Well-Being and Substitute Satisfaction

In varying degrees, most persons learn to associate food with interpersonal caring and affection, as well as with personal well-being. This learning begins with the earliest experiences of being fed as infants and continues through later pleasurable encounters with food. When food is readily available, food as a source of pleasure and satisfaction easily becomes functionally autonomous from basic nutritional need.

In addition, food readily provides a source of substitute satisfaction for emotional deprivation of various sorts. For example, the supply of affection, caring, and warmth from others may become depleted in disturbed interpersonal relationships. Self-regard and feelings of personal well-being may diminish in the wake of continuing life stress. For some individuals, dealing directly with such problems may be felt to be impossible, undesirable, or too difficult and disturbing. For them, eating may become an alternative course of action to problem solving, for it is an established resource for pleasure, the sense of well-being, and images of being loved and secure. As this behavioral response even temporarily moderates states of emotional deprivation, aloneness, and other dysphoric content, the tendency arises for the eating response to become increasingly independent of physiological need. In time, eating, instead of being responsive to nutritional need, may become a stimulus for further eating and form a self-sustaining autonomous system. Under such circumstances, the potential for overeating becomes high.

Thus, there are two distinct bases for the relative independence of eating from nutritional need. One is food as an intrinsic and symbolic source of well-being. Food tastes good; it symbolizes caring and security. We indulge. In this case, the problem of overeating requires reintegrating the individual's eating behavior with nutritional needs as defined in the individual's cultural setting.

The second basis for the separation of eating from nutritional need rests on food as a substitute source of satisfaction in situations where emotional deprivation and life stress of various sorts exist. The management of overeating, then, requires alteration in the way the individual copes with life's problems and stresses.

Overweight as Social Judgment

There is no *absolute* ideal weight range that can be established scientifically outside the context of a particular society or culture. "Overweight" is a relativistic concept defined by a given society (or culture) at a given period in its history. The "ideal range" of weight and body appearance reflects a complex of values and knowledge claims concerned with health, economics, aesthetics, and status.

Within a culture, there is generally a point where deviation in excess of the ideal weight range is labeled "overweight" or "obesity," just as deviation below this weight range is considered "underweight" or "emaciation." However, the point at which such judgments are made varies greatly from culture to culture. Thus, the clinical managment of an "overweight" problem for a self-referred

35-year-old Comanche Indian woman, living on tribal lands in the context of a culture that values fullness of body for women of her age, would differ substantially from the "overweight" problem of a self-referred 35-year-old Caucasian woman journalist working on an urban newspaper—even though both women live in the same country. There would be substantial differences not only in eating patterns and in the weight level judged as "overweight" in the two cases, but also in the ideal weight sought by each of the women.

THERAPEUTIC CONSIDERATIONS IN WEIGHT MANAGEMENT

Smoking and Eating as Hedonistic Experiences

Smoking and eating are both sources of considerable pleasure to the consumer. Each has become associated with behavior patterns that are embedded in a wide range of significant life functions. Often, they facilitate certain kinds of social interactions and enhance the events of which they are a part. The positive consequences associated with their occurrence are reinforcing, so that patterns of smoking and eating readily become firmly established as part of the individual's life style. The positive effects tend to be experienced as overbalancing the negatives that may also exist with both of these activities.

However, significant differences between these two pleasure-giving activities have implications for the therapeutic management of excessive indulgence. Life can proceed quite adequately without smoking—even better, according to medical judgment. Smoking unequivocally poses a health threat to many if not all individuals. When some toxic damage has occurred, the cessation of smoking may prevent further toxicity and may even permit the body to manage a substantial amount of reconstructive restitution. Even partial abstinence from smoking may permit anabolic changes to reduce the tissue injury that has resulted from smoking. Smoking is a behavior usually acquired in adolescence or early adulthood. The relaxation and social facilitation associated with smoking can be obtained through other behavioral alternatives.

Eating, on the other hand, is required for life. In addition to providing a source of pleasure, it is a necessary foundation for growth and health. Total abstinence from food is possible only for relatively brief periods of time without endangering the individual's existence.

Eating is not an acquired habit. It takes place at birth and is required throughout the life span. Even when quantities are reduced, or the nature of the food is changed, eating generally continues to be a pleasurable experience. There are no reasonable alternatives to eating.

The Energy-Balance Equation

The energy-balance equation states that a surplus of energy can occur only when the total intake exceeds the total expenditure. Energy intake can be approximated as the caloric value of ingested food, or, to be more precise, the caloric value of the actual amount of food assimilated by the cells of the body. The energy output is determined by the energy utilized by the body to sustain basic life processes plus that consumed in acting upon the environment. This thermodynamic equation presents the basic issue of overweight (i.e., storage of energy as fat), but offers only limited guidance to the clinical management of overeating. On the psychosocial level, the management of overeating involves a variety of factors, including the broad complexities of life style, habit patterns, and conflicting intrapsychic needs.

Hunger, Appetite, and the Glucostatic Regulatory Mechanism

The experience of being hungry seems to abate and even disappear early in the eating process, yet eating continues on the basis of appetite, social context, habit, and other factors. But most individuals who live in a food-affluent environment do not eat continuously. They experience a composite of internal and external stimuli that initiates their eating behavior and that is generally terminated far short of maximal capacity to ingest food.

Dr. Jean Mayer has postulated the existence of a central nervous system "hunger" center responsive to critical levels of blood sugar that can activate hunger sensations.[1] Eating results in the elevation of the blood sugar level to a point where a closely related center, the "satiety" center, is triggered off and the desire to eat is terminated. However, the elapsed time between the ingestion of food and the

1. J. Mayer. *Overweight: Causes, Costs, and Control.* Englewood Cliffs, New Jersey. Prentice-Hall, 1975.

transformation of the food into available blood sugars at a level that affects the satiety center is generally much longer than the time many people stop eating. There are some people whose behavior strongly suggests an effective internal "stop-eating" trigger, but for others, external factors seem to be much more dominant determinants of the amount and duration of eating.

Research on the selective breeding of strains of "fat" and "lean" mice support the probable existence of genetic factors in some conditions of obesity. The two strains of mice eat to different weight-level plateaus when they are placed in an *ad libitum*, food-affluent environment. However, even the "fat" mice stop eating at some point and maintain their relative weight and size gain at a fairly stable level unless some surgical or environmental intervention is introduced. Similar effects have been noted in rats through laboratory-induced brain lesions or disease-caused lesions; that is, body weight rises sharply to a new plateau. Thus, the trigger mechanism for hunger and satiety may exist at different levels on the basis of genetic variation, traumatic intrusion, or other factors that may set limits of weight in a food-affluent environment.

It is probable that similar physiological regulators exist in humans. However, developmental conditioning and psychosocial factors associated with the eating situation may readily override the effects of these regulators in the determination of eating behavior. Clinically, it is well known that the overeater who has been physiologically satiated and who may even report being absolutely stuffed may begin eating again almost immediately if a particularly appetizing food, a particular social facilitation, or a stress-related stimulus for eating should occur.

The therapeutic implications of research thus far are that psychosocial determinants are far more important for the management of overeating than are physiological cues. Perhaps, by altering eating patterns, the individual may become more responsive to internal states of hunger and fullness, in which case the effect of these weak physiological regulators would become more relevant.

EVALUATING AN INDIVIDUAL'S WEIGHT-MANAGEMENT NEEDS

It is suggested that an effective weight-management program for a particular individual include the following four components, in addition to the therapeutic relationship: (1) a medical history and assessment of physical status; (2) a psychosocial history of experiences related to eating; (3) a "nutritional intake and circumstances of eating" (NICE) diary; and (4) an exercise diary.

These four components provide a broad base for planning a diet, developing an exercise regimen, setting a range of tolerable weight changes, and establishing psychotherapeutic interventions that will facilitate change in eating behavior and stress management. A brief elaboration of the four components is given below. This is followed by consideration of psychotherapeutic (hypnotherapeutic) interventions as part of the total weight-reduction program.

Medical History and Physical Status

Thyroxin insufficiency, gastrointestinal disease, and cardiovascular dysfunction are but a few of the conditions that may affect the nutritional-input–energy-output balance and lead to weight increase. The medical history, physical examination, metabolic evaluation, and determination of endocrine function provide an understanding of physiological needs that may be relevant to the individual's weight. Thus, insulin, thyroxin, cardiovascular medication, or some other physiological agent may be helpful and even necessary to the program of weight reduction.

Psychosocial History Related to Eating

A careful review of experiences related to food and eating, with an emphasis upon the individual's prior efforts to manage the weight problem, emotional reactions to body weight, self-image implications of both "overweight" and "loss of weight," and life circumstances relevant to body weight and eating behaviors, helps in uncovering important psychosocial factors that need to be considered in the weight-reduction program. The client can provide much of this information by completing a questionnaire, following which an interview can be used to explore the written report further. Questions such as the following can then be clarified:

1. *Motivational aspects*: What motivated the person in previous attempts to lose weight? Who supported, discouraged, or affected the

effort? Have there been changes in motivation over time? Does the person believe in the possibility of change?

2. *Self-image effects*: What view of the self did the person have at the beginning and end of each cycle of weight gain and loss? What is the curent view of self? What is the person's general attitude toward life?

3. *Management aspects*: What worked to control food intake and energy output? What was the maximum total weight change? Were there any notable events associated with decontrol? How long did the cycle of weight loss and weight gain take? What stresses were active at the time of weight gain and loss? Did weight loss lead to disturbances in general coping capabilities?

The encouraging therapist tends to emphasize the learning derived from the analysis of the previous motivations, self-image perceptions, and control procedures. Much can also be learned from an understanding of the factors that led to decontrol and the problems that appear to need solution because of their previous counterproductive effects. The client's new weight-management program is interpreted as evidence of determination and continued belief in the realistic possibility of maintaining long-term weight reduction.

The pessimistic therapist tends to view the client's cycles of weight loss followed by weight gain as foreboding failure—as strong evidence of the client's unwillingness or inability to make a commitment to a lifelong revised pattern of eating and energy output. Concern may be expressed about the potential negative consequences of another failure experience in weight management. The client's readiness to repeat the same cycle may be viewed as an unrealistic appraisal of past experiences, as well as a *sub rosa* attack upon his or her self-esteem.

There are some individuals for whom the loss of a significant amount of weight, with its accompanying changes in body configuration, may become a psychological threat to their coping capacity. The weight loss may become a destabilizing factor that precipitates mood dyphoria, thought disturbances, or other serious dysfunctions. The psychosocial chronology of previous weight-management attempts serves an important diagnostic function in providing clues to such potentially disruptive reactions. Thus, the management of weight reduction may in some cases have to proceed concurrently with extensive psychotherapy for personality disturbances, or else weight reduction may have to be deferred until the client has achieved a more general capacity for coping with the exigencies of living.

The NICE (Nutritional Intake and Circumstances of Eating) Diary

Behavioral records of eating patterns and the circumstances surrounding each incident of food ingestion have proven to be of considerable clinical value in assessing weight-management needs and in planning the individual diet program. The client records every eating incident for two weeks, indicating the time the incident occurred, the food and amount eaten, its taste, and the associated feelings and circumstances. The diary provides the client and therapist with a client-generated data base about eating habits. It serves to heighten the client's awareness of the internal and external cues associated with the act of eating, the emotional reactions to eating, and the total caloric intake.

Some client resistance to the NICE record keeping is to be expected; the time factor involved is the reason most frequently given. For many clients, this stated reason shields the discomfort that is generated when they are confronted with the hard reality of their own eating habits. Failure to make entries is a common manifestation of the tendency to avoid facing the amount of calories ingested. The therapist should discuss the client's complaints and show understanding of the discomfort that is being experienced. There should be confident assurances, however, about the value of the NICE diary for the planning of the individual program.

By having to make a public record to be shared with the therapist, clients become sensitized to their feelings surrounding eating and their particular pattern of postprandial remorse. They become aware that this self-recrimination, coming as it does while they are still enjoying the experience of eating, serves to remove inhibition about later eating. They begin to understand that the expiation has rather painlessly reduced whatever guilt, shame, or sin may have been associated with the eating. For many clients, this heightened awareness may also be one of their first experiences in acting as "cotherapists" in responsibly sharing the management of their weight problem.

The Exercise Record

The pedometer is a simple mechanical device that yields a rough record of how much walking the client has done during the day. The inclusion of this figure, plus a record of the kind and duration of any additional exercise in the NICE diary, provides a useful base line of energy output. The two-week sample of energy input through food and energy output through exercise graphically displays the existing nutritional surplus that is stored as fat. The client has a self-generated index that helps in understanding one aspect of weight accumulation. Furthermore, the objective pedometer readings provide a basis for graduated increases in energy output through walking, supplemented by other exercise—a base that is not dependent upon memory and impressions of action. The decision to increase physical exercise contributes to the individual's sense of control over self in a way comparable to that resulting from deliberate action by the individual to moderate his or her patterns of eating.

THE HYPNOTHERAPY OF OVEREATING

The multidimensional evaluation necessary for an adequate program of weight management embodies the following convictions: (1) The existing health status of the client should be protected; (2) a weight-management program should be adapted to the client's capacity for change; and (3) the maintenance of change in body weight for the long term should be a prime consideration in selecting a weight-reduction strategy. In accordance with these convictions, a weight-management program involves a multifaceted approach that may include dietary regimen, medical intervention, exercise, self-help (e.g, bibliotherapy), self-help groups and social support networks, stress-reduction procedures, psychotherapy, and hypnotherapy.

The following discussion focuses on altering patterns of eating behavior. In essence, the goal is to modify the enjoyment associated with overeating. Particular attention is given to the contributions of hypnotherapy to the processes of expediting and sustaining changes in eating behavior.

Initial Hypnotherapeutic Experiences: Example of Determining Weight-Control Readiness and First Goal

The psychotherapist who uses hypnotherapy in the program of weight management tends to be perceived by even psychologically sophisticated clients as beings possessed of therapeutic techniques that will relieve the clients of almost all responsibility for self-control and involvement in the management of their weight problems. Overtly or covertly, such a client has a hypnosis fantasy wherein an omniscient, ever-present benign monitoring force obliges the person to observe positive eating practices; this force is thought of as preventing harmful dietary transgressions while permitting the essence of pleasure in the eating situation to be retained—the best of all possible worlds!

No matter how divergent this fantasy may be from the world of hypnotic realities, it often revives the client's hope for a successful outcome of weight management and serves as a catalyst for facilitating the person's readiness to alter patterns of eating. Thus, the clinician has a delicate balancing task: to sustain the motivation for therapy and readiness to change that this hypnosis fantasy energizes, while at the same time persuading the client to participate as cotherapist and to become deeply involved in the program of change. The broad-spectrum diagnostic evaluation is a valuable help in this connection. Its procedures communicate to the client that the therapist conceives of the weight-management program as a multidimensional approach involving the active participation of the client, even though the hypnosis fantasy is not overtly challenged.

Early in the therapeutic relationship, the therapist acknowledges the potency of the hypnosis fantasy. In the second or third therapeutic session, even if the diagnostic evaluation is still in progress, the client is taught self-hypnosis—that is, how to enter into trance and use hypnosis to lower tension, and how to begin the exploration of inner psychological space. The relaxation aspect is emphasized not only as a means of dealing with some of the tensions associated with any serious effort to change well-established pleasure-producing habits, but also as a pathway for experiencing other hynotherapeutic learning.

The second hypnotherapy orienting experience is through the use of the Chevreul pendulum or finger signaling (see Chapter 2, pp. 29–31). The ideometer procedure permits exploring with the client covert attitudes toward the program of weight management, especially with regard to required changes in eating practices. To help insure success, an initial weight goal is set at a realistic level. Once this goal is achieved, a maintenance period of two to four months is used to sustain the weight level. This successful experience then becomes the basis for another round of weight reduction and weight maintenance until the desired weight is obtained. Repeated success with these successive rounds help to insure lifelong changes in the pattern of eating behavior.

The client in the following example was a 38 year-old male auto mechanic shop foreman, whose weight of 295 pounds was interfering with his work performance. His history of overweight began during adolescence, with regular gains of three to five pounds each year except for two intervals: one for three years while in military service (when he was aged 21–24), and the second for two years after his marriage (when he was aged 27–29). He had been through at least four cycles of losing weight—the maximum weight loss being 50 pounds at one try—but had regained his original weight plus an added five to eight pounds following the regimen. The interaction below occurred during the third therapy session:

THERAPIST: The inner part of your mind has indicated its "yes," "no," "I don't know," and "I do not want to answer" signals with the pendulum . . . What is the first question you would like to ask the inner part of your mind?

CLIENT: I've told you that I've tried several systems. Each system worked for a while, but then I ended up heavier than I was at the beginning. So I would like to know if hypnosis will help.

T: Let's ask the inner part of your mind to free itself from your conscious hopes and wishes and to look deep inside yourself. Does J. R. [the client] have a really good chance to use hypnosis successfully in this new effort at long-term weight management?

[The pendulum remains absolutely stationary for ten to fifteen seconds. Then, very slowly, it begins a clockwise motion, which is the "I don't know" signal, but shortly thereafter switches into the "yes" mode. The therapist remains silent, suggesting by his silence that more might happen. Gradually, the "yes" response strengthens and swings more vigorously. The client, watching the motion with fascination, begins to smile broadly.]

T: How would you interpret this response?

C: I guess this part of my mind was really looking around. I really wondered about that "I don't know" answer and felt really good when that "yes" answer turned up.

T: I agree with you . . . I would read it that the inner part of your mind remains basically hopeful about the future and is willing to continue working for a way to reach your goals. You remember our discussion of successive periods of weight management: first a weight goal and success in reaching it, then a maintenance period followed by a new round . . . What should the first weight goal be?

C: I would really like to get down to 200 pounds as the first goal.

T: Well, let's check with the inner part of your mind . . . Would the goal of 200 pounds be a good first goal? [The pendulum quickly responds with a "no" signal. Then the therapist stabilizes the pendulum.] Should the weight goal be less than 200 pounds? ["No" signal.] More than 200 pounds? ["Yes" signal.]

Let me ask the inner part of your mind to indicate its judgments as I move along by ten-pound increments as to the first weight goal. What about getting down to 210 pounds? ["No."] 220? ["No."] 230? ["No."] 240? ["No."] 250? ["Yes."]

[The client is totally absorbed by the pendulum, watching it as though it is in someone else's hand, exercising its own decision. He is impressed by the precision of this inner voice that is indicating a weight goal of forty-five pounds below his present weight, slightly below the maximum weight reduction previously achieved.]

T: Does the inner part of your mind feel secure that it can help you to maintain this new weight level for four months before you start your next round? [An immediate definite "yes" movement of the pendulum occurs.] Is the inner part of your mind ready to help you change your pattern of eating permanently? [The pendulum response is "I do not choose to answer."] That's interesting. What do you think that means?

C: I guess that deep inside of me there is still an unsureness about the long haul.

T: Let me ask the inner part of your mind if it would support a change in your eating habits for the next six months? [The "yes" response appears very quickly.] Does the inner part of your mind know of any reason why you should not start on your weight-management program? [The "no" response quickly appears.]

This client's experience demonstrates how the Chevreul pendulum questioning explores areas of ambivalence and uncertainty, heightens the client's awareness of his or her own psychological complexity; taps to some degree the client's hypnosis fantasy for motivational support for the treatment; and emphasizes self-responsibility, long-term goals, and continual "check-back" with the client for individualization of the program.

In Chapter 11, six strategies are presented for altering the hedonistic smoking experience. The multitude of therapeutic procedures reported in the literature to modify eating habits can also be classified under one or more of these strategies. The value of this classification is twofold: First, the clinician can develop innovative, individualized programs of psychotherapy designed to meet the special needs of particular clients; and, second, the classification provides a basis for recognizing a new strategy when it does appear on the scene.

The Strategy of Future Positive Consequences

Obese individuals who seek psychological help are concerned about the consequences of their weight in terms of their health, the social acceptability of their appearance, the flexibility of their physical movements, and their own self-esteem. The therapeutic strategy of future positive consequences emphasizes the achievability of future goals as the patterns of eating change. There is a mobilization of fantasy, imagery, and hope centered about this projected better future state. The hypnotic-trance state of consciousness serves as an excellent therapeutic medium for the intensification of these fantasies. Auto-hypnotic exercises provide many opportunities for the progressive reshaping of the individual's perception of self, and for acceptance of the approaching new self-image.

Dr. Herbert Spiegel's method for the control of smoking (see Chapter 11, 178–179) emphasizes the positive consequences for health and the quality of life in becoming a nonsmoker. Central importance is also placed upon the individual's self-reinforcement of messages about three life-sustaining values of nonsmoking while in hypnotic trance: "Smoking is a poison for my body;" "I need my body in order to live;" and "I owe my body respect and protection." The prescribed requirement for scheduled repetition of the exercise (ten times per day) means that a need for a decision about whether or not to smoke is never far in time from an exercise experience, especially during the early stages of transition in one's identity from "smoker" to "non-smoker."

With only minor modifications, the Spiegel approach can be effectively adapted to the transition from "overeater" to "balanced eater." At this stage of treatment, the client has already had some basic experience with the use of hypnotic trance for relaxation and stress reduction. The training session in which the Spiegel procedure is practiced during hypnotic trance is recorded so that the client can use the tape, as needed, for achieving mastery of the exercise. The eating-related value statements are "Overeating is a threat to my body and my life expectancy;" "I need a healthy body to enjoy and sustain life;" and "I owe my body respect and protection through balanced eating."

This exercise is presented to the overweight client in the context that the decision to eat or not to eat is the client's prerogative. The purpose of the exercise is to help those clients who want to sustain their decision to become balanced eaters and achieve a new weight status for themselves. The prescribed practice is regarded as essential, to be followed as strictly as one would a schedule for taking an important health-restoring medication.

The client who is overweight has learned to feel quite conscious about the physical self, most often with an accompanying self-devaluative attitude. The hope for changes in body configuration that would permit, for example, comfort in wearing a swim suit, can be an intrinsic part of the motivation that sustains the patient on a weight-reduction regimen. The pleasurable anticipation of a socially approved body weight, as well as the concurrent expansion of physical functioning, are future positive consequences that counterbalance the loss of immediate gratification that comes with decreased food intake.

Clinicians who have worked with weight-dysphoric clients have incorporated these hopes for the future into their therapeutic practices. For example, a client may be encouraged to purchase an unusually fine garment—one considerably more expensive than he or she would usually buy, and one that will fit when the new weight level has been achieved. During relaxed trance, the client is encouraged to fantasize wearing the garment, enjoying its fit, getting the socially positive feedback he or she has been wanting. The client is encouraged to describe feelings in detail, to vividly experience growth in self-esteem, and to believe in the realistic possibilities of this future becoming part of the ongoing present. The procedure blends the contemporary reality of the garment as a concrete symbol of personal commitment to weight reduction with the future positive consequences experienced by a fantasy sampling of the goal area.

The suggestion has also been made that a client who is overweight find a photograph of himself or herself in which the body shape is pleasing. If such is not available, the client is instructed to look through magazines or other sources for a picture of a body configuration that is reasonably close to where the client wants to be when "maintenance" eating begins. This picture is then cut out, and a photograph of the client's own head is affixed to the target image. The client focuses upon this target configuration as a future goal. Hypnotic trance enhances the vividness of the future-time fantasies of this new physical self functioning in significant life situations, and helps the client to sample the future consequences of continued balanced eating. These vivid fantasies serve to sustain motivation by clarifying the goals toward which the client is moving, and by contributing to the client's confidence and self-esteem.

Fantasies of the future serve an additional function quite apart from motivational enhancement. The client may signal areas of potential stress that may be associated with successful changes in eating habits and altered weight status. When such dissonances appear, whether they be in potential sexual functioning, interpersonal relations, or whatever, they merit careful therapeutic attention if the program of balanced eating is to be maintained. Since the client is also encouraged to pursue these fantasy explorations on his or her own, the same attention must also be given to "red-flag" fantasies of distress when these are reported back to the therapist.

The Strategy of Negative Accentuation:
Example of Vivifying the Negative during Trance

The psychotherapeutic strategy of negative accentuation addresses itself directly to the ambivalent state that has brought the overweight client to the therapeutic setting. The hedonistic aspect of overeating, evident in such reports as "It tastes so good," or "It make me feel so satisfied and contented to feel that chocolate milk slide down my throat." would never bring the overeating client to search for help. Rather, the substantial negative effects of sustained overeating—those that pertain to the present as well as to the fear of future consequences—are the ones that motivate the client to explore changes in eating patterns.

In the case of cigarette smoking, the physical consequences may take years to become manifest in pulmonary and cardiovascular symptoms. Overeating, on the other hand, manifests itself fairly quickly in increased size and weight when caloric intake is substantially greater than caloric utilization. As the individual's volume increases, often without a relative corresponding increase in striated musculature, even minor exertions may become accompanied by huffing and puffing.

Clothing ceases to fit, and ready fatigue becomes a familiar experience to the individual carrying around an additional 50 or more pounds. Then there are the pressures of social conformity when one views oneself in the mirror or becomes aware of the group's attitudes toward the fat. These negative experiences may either be acknowledged or denied, but once a person comes for therapy, it is reasonable to assume that the negative awarenesses have not been sufficient by themselves to modify the client's eating behavior.

In applying the strategy of negative accentuation, the client is asked to prepare a list of personally negative consequences of overeating and to rank them in order of increasing negative value. From this list, the client chooses the first one(s) to work with. This procedure emphasizes the cotherapist responsibilities of the client in the management of the program of eating control, and also provides a guide for fantasy exercises for additional negative accentuation.

Even though the client is the person who prepares the list of negative effects and chooses the one(s) to be initially elaborated, it remains prudent for the therapist to use either the Chevreul pendulum or the finger-signaling technique to check whether accentuating the negative in fantasy would be acceptable to the client. An affirmative response confirms the client's readiness to accept the heightened stress that may be associated with negative accentuation during hypnotic trance. It also implies that the client recognizes the purpose of negative accentuation in facilitating better self-management of eating.

The particular client in the following demonstration was a 45-year-old male who had drawn up a list of negative consequences of overeating that began with a double chin and ended with a very deep concern about high blood pressure and diabetes, both of which were quite frequent on his father's side of the family. He had always had a vigorous appetite, but his wieght problem had become aggravated since he had become sales manager of an insurance firm, a position that required frequent luncheon and dinner meetings with clients. He had gained 25 pounds in the past nine months, reaching his present weight of 230 pounds. There was a classical history of crash diets and rapid regaining of weight, usually to a point greater than the preceding figure. This time he had made a commitment to his family to stay with the program under the supervision of his internist and psychotherapist. His only constraint was that no appetite-suppressing medication be used.

Four psychotherapy sessions in which hypnosis was used for training in relaxation and imagery production preceded the following interaction:

THERAPIST: You listed your double chin, tight clothes, and having to bend over to see your toes as your first three negative consequences.

CLIENT: The three of them really belong to a common feeling of being bloated. Like a balloon that was shaped like a human figure but then became distorted because too much air was pumped into it. I have begun to feel like parts of me are becoming exaggerated in size—unreal.

T: It must be really uncomfortable for you to feel that parts of you feel unreal, almost alien to yourself. You indicated with the Chevreul pendulum that you were ready to give full emphasis to these feelings while in trance so that the inner part of your mind could get the message to use them to become a balanced eater.

Please raise your right hand in front of you with the palm facing away, and focus upon your fingers as you have done several times before. Let the feelings of heaviness come into your hand as your eyes maintain their fixed focus . . . As you feel your hand moving down, let the heaviness in your eyes increase until they want to close . . . Good . . . Let them close and let your arm come to rest in your lap . . . Letting go . . . your whole being relaxing . . . drifting . . . drifting . . . drifting to an eating situation where you have an inexhaustible supply of food in front of you . . . Signal with your right index finger when that image or that idea is clear to you. . . .

Okay . . . [Dissociation is suggested:] I'm going to ask you to describe the scene, and as you talk you become more and more involved in the scene until part of you feels like it is right there in the scene and the main part remains right here with me watching what is happening. . . .

C: I see myself in the restaurant . . . There is a huge smorgasbord table spread out in front of me piled high with wonderful food . . . It all looks and smells so appetizing. . . .

T: Imagine yourself with an unlimited appetite . . . Begin feeding yourself from the heaping plates . . . and imagine that it is like time-lapse photography . . . As the food goes into you . . . it is processed almost immediately . . . and you can see the effects of the food . . . as if weeks and weeks of eating were being condensed into minutes. . . .

C: I can taste the food on the back of my tongue and just feel the swallowing . . . The skin under my chin is filling out . . . It seems to be getting larger and fuller until my chin seems to blend into this under-skin . . . I can hardly see the neck line . . . It looks almost like a frog's neck, and my head is forced upward a way by the mass under my skin . . . That's really weird-looking. . . .

T: Keep on with your eating . . . See where your image leads you as you continue eating. . . .

C: Now I see myself beginning to get larger around my chest and middle . . . A funny thing is happening . . . Now I can see myself only from the back, and I am no longer sitting on a chair but on a bench, and my back end is beginning to drape over it . . . I see the midseam in the back of my jacket pulling apart . . . as though it might give way any moment . . . Now it shifts again and I am looking at the front of me . . . I can hardly recognize myself . . . My eyes are deep in my head with big rolls of cheek. . . .

T: How are you feeling?

C: Terrible . . . Yet I still see myself eating . . . and getting more and more bloated . . . hardly a large enough opening in my face for the food to be put in . . . I don't know if I could stand up on my legs if I tried. . . .

T: Intensify the image . . . [Client comanagement is suggested:] Bring it to the point where it will be most helpful to you in managing your daily eating program. . . .

C: I'm beginning to get a sickish feeling inside . . . That's hardly human . . . I can't seem to recognize myself . . . It stopped feeding itself. . . .

T: Good . . . Make use of this image when your inner mind needs it to help you become a balanced eater . . . Now condense future time . . . See that image begin to restore itself as the eating becomes a balanced eating . . . When the figure of yourself is back to where it pleases you . . . signal with your right index finger . . . Count yourself back to the here and now. . . .

The preceding example illustrates how personally negative consequences of over-eating can be vivified during trance. There is yet another way in which the strategy of negative accentuation can be used. In this case, the therapist helps to transform what would have been an enticing eating experience for the client during trance to one that is highly negative by introducing an aversive element that had been suggested earlier by the client.

Prior to the hypnotic trance, the client is asked to rank several food and eating situations that have particularly compelling visual, olfactory, or social cues that heighten the attractiveness of the food and increase the urgency of the need to eat. As vividly as possible, the client describes in detail what gives this food its particular potency—its appearance, aroma, taste, texture, and so forth. The client also proposes a dysphoric element that would make the food or the eating situation completely negative. The Chevreul pendulum or the finger-signaling method is used to obtain consent to proceed with hypnosis. A self-induced trance can be used by the client to elaborate the very compelling positive food situation described in the waking state. The client is encouraged to enhance the food imagery as fully as possible, to the point where consumption is eagerly anticipated. Then the client-selected dysphoric element is introduced.

One client had elaborated the fragrance, marbled coloration, and texture of a highly prized imported French cheese when the suggestion was made that he see it covered with the maggots he had mentioned. His face registered his disgust. In his imagery, he looked around the room, and no one else seemed to be aware of the maggots on this cheese. The others were sampling it with apparent relish. With grim determination, and while still in trance, he decided to put a wedge of cheese on a cracker and place it in his mouth with eyes closed. The sensation of movement in his mouth created a disgust and nausea he could not control. He began gagging and dry-heaving. He "emptied" his mouth into his handkerchief while the therapist encouraged him to maintain the sensations until he felt that they had registered on his inner mind. Then he was asked to come back to the here and now and allow his insides to settle down. The same exercise was repeated three times at this session before going on to the next item on his list.

During the last trial, the therapist emphasized to the client that the particular aversive reactions to the specific foods would not automatically occur whenever he encountered the food or the food situation. However, if he decided that he did not want to yield to the compelling force of the food, then all he needed to do was close his eyes and count to three, and the vividness of the maggots would be there. As long as he was the one to make decision, the effectiveness of the maggot image would continue. Then he would open his eyes and congratulate himself for his control over this food compulsion.

Only a small number of clients who overeat are able or willing to evoke such a strong aversive image with respect to a specially cherished food. However, even a modest decrease in attractive mental imagery provides an opportunity to mobilize other control mechanisms. It is clear that guilt, shame, and a host of other feelings may be used to reduce the positive valence of food.

The strategy of accentuating the negative by aversive associations to a particular food or food situation requires that the client be assured that the aversion does not spread to food in general. Since the appetite of the overeater is relatively independent of nutritional needs of the body, most often the desire to eat is evoked by physical or social environmental stimuli associated with a particular food or food situation. The strategy is especially useful for those clients who, early in the therapeutic program, report overwhelming impulses to eat certain foods or to eat in certain food situations.

The Strategy of Alternative Means of Gratification

The psychotherapeutic strategy of alternative means of gratification acknowledges the broad spectrum of important human functions that are intimately associated with food and eating. These functions are briefly surveyed at the beginning of this chapter in the discussion of the place of food in the human experience. Love, security, social acceptance, religious worship, and reduction of tension are all part of the eating experience. More needs than the body's nutritional ones are obviously gratified by eating. For many people who overeat, the pressure to gratify these needs through eating may overshadow their nutritional needs. When the satisfaction that comes with eating has resulted primarily from reducing tension, experiencing love and caring via food, or sensing the security of a full abdomen, then eating as a response to nutritional needs becomes very much attenuated.

The strategy of alternative means of gratification involves two kinds of reorientation of goals and means. One requires that the therapist and client identify the non-nutritional needs that have heretofore led to overeating so that the client can be helped to learn more direct, noncaloric ways of satisfying them. The other requires that the nutritional aspect of eating be given a new emphasis based on the recognition that gratification related to body needs is *qualitatively* different from the "*quantitative* gratification" orientated toward the non-nutritional needs of the individual.

The detailed two-week NICE diary (see p. 206) serves as a valuable data source for helping the client to identify the specific conditions of time, place, and circumstance that generate the inner tensions and stresses leading to non-nutritional eating. Awareness of these conditions enables the client to make use of the hypnotic state of trance consciousness as a medium for developing relaxation and release of tension. Then, whether in trance or out of trance, the client is in a better position to explore ways to alter the conditions creating these particular stresses and to develop new approaches to fulfill non-nutritional needs.

However, even when the client begins to discriminate between eating to meet nutritional needs and eating to gratify other needs, and even when progress toward satisfying the latter more directly is being made during the course of psychotherapy, poor eating habits reinforced over hundreds of repetitions are likely to remain, especially the habit of "quantitative gratification." Sensory cues (appearance, aroma, etc.) are of clear importance in stimulating the overeater's mental imagery to begin the eating process. Once ingestion occurs, it is as if the process becomes autonomous, independent of the usual influence of physiological regulatory mechanisms except for the sensation of fullness. Behaviorally, the overeater eats rapidly, progressing through the available food supply in a determined and inexorable fashion, giving the impression that there is only minor awareness of the specific differences between foods. It seems as if the goal of filling the empty space within as a prerequisite for a sense of well-being has shunted other considerations and physiological sensations away from consciousness, leaving only the habitual "quantitative gratification" guide to eating with its inevitable caloric overload.

The shift to the alternative "qualitative gratification" for eating is a requisite step in progress toward the restoration or establishment of control over the eating process. Paradoxically, the overeater needs to become more *aware* of what he or she is eating during the actual eating process—to become responsive to the specific characteristics of each bite of food. Involvement with each bite of food creates the needed deceleration of the eating pace, which in turn allows time for the body's more subtle physiological responses to become apparent to the individual. Finally, food as a nutritional value, a goal in its own right, rather than food and eating as instrumentalities serving to satisfy other needs, must come to be appreciated. Almost all bariatric therapists place emphasis upon the nutritional value of food as part of re-educating the eating process that a balanced eater learns to traverse.

Obviously, the food being eaten must be attended to if heightened consciousness about different properties and sensations is to develop. The portion contained on the eating utensil must be seen if its visual identity is to become differentiated; it must be looked at before being deposited into the open mouth—and looking at the food means that the gaze is not directed at a book, a TV screen, or some other object. Attention is focused upon the appearance and aroma of the food. Then, after it is placed in the mouth, taste and texture definition cannot occur if gulping or swallowing occurs immediately. Therefore, it needs to remain in the mouth—savored, tasted, chewed for texture, enhanced with saliva, dissolved, and experienced before swallowing. Finally, the residual taste experience in the mouth needs to be noticed before the next mouthful is taken.

Several purposes are served by a pattern of eating that stresses the qualitative character of the food: (1) The unit of food becomes psychologically defined as the spoonful, not the portion or the plate; (2) there is a qualitative encounter with the food that emphasizes its pleasurable and aesthetic quality, rather than its space-filling function; and (3) the differentiation of the eating process into substeps acts to decelerate the pace of eating.

Hypnotic trance can be most helpful to some clients in learning to adapt to the new mode of eating. The client is encouraged to self-induce trance at the beginning of each meal. Specific self-suggestions are, of course, fitted to the particular client's needs and circumstances. However, the following four suggestions, offered by the therapist, indicate the basic concepts that are emphasized:

1. "This new way of eating will be rewarding to you in many more ways than your old habits. You will come to have more control over what you eat and how much you eat. You will enjoy what you eat because you will be aware of what you are eating. The decreased caloric intake will help you to be more at peace with yourself."

2. "You can be relaxed while you are eating because now you are gratifying basic nutritional needs, not some other hidden agendas. Those other needs can be dealt with more directly. You know that there is no nutritional crisis that demands urgent action."

3. "Tune in on all the nuances of flavor, aroma, texture. Use your trance to enjoy your food. Discover how less food can be fully satisfying."

4. "Your new eating habits will give your body time to signal when you have had enough to eat. You can stop eating whenever your appetite control says enough, even in the middle of a mouthful."

The therapy of overeating, in the judgment of most clinicians, requires a reduced pace of eating. Many timing devices have been suggested: for example, the metronome, the commercial variable time beeper that signals each mouthful, the counting of chews before swallowing, the placement of the eating utensils on the table between mouthfuls, and so forth. Each method has merit for some persons, especially those who need external supports for learning self-regulation in the early phases of their program.

The Strategy of Conscious Decision

It is the client's right to be able to choose freely whether or not to overeat. The purposes of the psychotherapeutic strategy of conscious control are to protect the client's freedom to make choices, to assure the client that in each eating situation he or she will have such a choice *before* the food has been eaten, and to reduce the occasions when the client experiences awareness only *after* the food has been partially or wholly consumed. Such belated awareness is very close to the experience of the smoker who is drawing deeply on a cigarette without being aware of having made a decision to smoke.

The overeater's self-report of such incidents is also strongly reminiscent of the experience of the sleepwalker who suddenly wakens to find himself or herself somewhere upon life's highway instead of securely asleep at home in bed. As with the sleepwalker, the late hours of evening and the wee hours of night seem to be the bewitching times for the overeater. The particular person may seem to be busy at the workbench or the study desk, or to be sitting engrossed in an easy chair in front of the TV. Yet at some point, it is as if some inner power disengages the individual from the setting and moves him or her over to a known food repository (refrigerator, food bin, etc.) where food is selected; avid eating then begins, either *in situ* or where the individual had been engaged. Then at some point, the overeater seems to become aware of the half-full bowl of food, the empty peanut jar, or the sandwich remnant in the dish. The process may even have involved complex preparation. Again, the client's self-report makes it appear as if some dissociation of self takes place in response to an inner craving that leads the client to proceed to the food source and satisfy the inner need to eat without involving the total person. Of course, there also are many visits to the refrigerator or the food storage bin that are eagerly anticipated and carried out in full consciousness, only to have the usual self-recriminations occur after satisfaction.

A similar affective quality to that experienced in dissociation is seen in the type of overeater activity at parties or other occasions when ample supplies of food are available, seemingly widely distributed in trays on tables, sideboards, and everywhere. Apparently the food is *always within arm's reach*, no matter where one is in the room—or so it seems from the overeater's perspective. Actually, the overeater is seen to maintain a regular migration that brings him or her close to the food: The person engages in conversation with people near the food, admires a painting or an art object adjoining food trays, sits in a chair near the loaded coffee table, or otherwise places the body so that a continuous stream of hand-to-mouth food maneuvers is quite easy. Yet, if questioned after the event, the overeater will focus upon social participation, with relatively little awareness of the continuous self-feeding—an instance of the kind of disengagement of self reminiscent of some night-time snacking.

The hypnotherapeutic procedure for the strategy of conscious decision about eating follows the same pattern as that described for smoking in Chapter 11. The client learns to "freeze" arm action at a point where the food approaches the mouth, as with the cigarette. The client has a clear understanding that the "freeze" action is not meant to pre-empt the client's decision-making prerogative, but only to bring the decision making to the conscious level. Before the arm is freed, the client goes through a review of the health-values exercise (the modified Spiegel technique), and then the arm is free to move. The client has had the opportunity to make a responsible choice. The specifics of these "freeze" experiences will be dependent upon the particular settings and circumstances in which a given client experiences these bypasses of a decision to eat.

There are instances of unconscious snacking during a dissociative state where awareness of the forbidden indulgence does not spontaneously occur, not even after the snacking is over. Such a case is reported in Chapter 8. The "secret eater" in this case was enabled to make a conscious decision about eating, once she was provided with the shocking evidence of her unconscious food behavior during a posthypnotically induced conflict designed to point up her specific problem. It would be well to review the demonstration (see pp. 123–128) at this time.

The Strategy of Environmental Change

Of considerable importance for progress in the shift of identity from "overeater" to "balanced eater" is the impact of environmental conditions related to the eating behaviors. The modification of many of these environmental conditions can offer considerable support for the new "balanced-eater" practices. The fact that being a balanced eater requires lifelong changes in eating habits has low attractiveness to those overeaters who continue to seek short-term "crash" programs that will dissolve their weight problems without requiring uncomfortable or radical changes in either eating behavior or environmental circumstances. Unfortunately, even short-term results tend to be inherently disappointing because the participants soon return to their pre-existing patterns of eating without having changed any of the environmental conditions that supported the original overeating.

Clinical studies of weight-maintenance programs in which clients have sustained weight changes over significant time periods make it abundantly clear that environmental changes are essential components that support such outcomes. The accurate weighing scale is one such environmental factor that is consistently rated high in most studies of sustained maintenance. Frequent weighings with a careful recording of all readings seem to support one's efforts by providing an objective record of something happening—a record that is relatively less subject to wish distortion. Also, the use of smaller serving dishes is recommended as perceptually more consonant with smaller-sized portions, in contrast to modest-sized amounts resting on a larger expanse of space. Some overeaters give considerable merit to the purchase of a uniquely personal table setting to serve as a symbolic reminder of their resolve to become balanced eaters. Another highly useful environmental controlling condition is preparing a carefully thought-out shopping list prior to setting out for the market place, and strictly observing the list, dutifully resisting impulse buying and overpurchasing—two practices commonly observed as the overeater wanders through the aisles of the food market. The prepared list not only guides the purchase of the kinds and amounts of food, but also provides a "success" experience for the purchaser for not having yielded to impulse buying.

In general, the studies seem to favor regular times for meals (including snacks), with multiple small eating episodes rather than a few large meals. Night-time eating represents a difficult problem for many overeaters. There are three general environmental controls that can be activated: (1) placing a strict limit on the kinds and the amounts of food available in the usual food repositories (refrigerator, pantry, hidden storage areas); (2) creating difficulties in access to the food through the use of locks, bolts, and the like, with the keys entrusted to someone else; and (3) placing red flags on the refrigerator door or providing other psychological barriers between the food and the overeater. The individual has to try one or more of these approaches to discover what actually is helpful.

The environmental setting in which food is eaten needs to be differentiated from settings in which other activities occur that may deflect awareness from the food and thus bypass the controlled eating process. The chair by the TV set, the study or work desk, the bridge table, the bed, and the refrigerator need to be defined as places where eating does not take place, no matter what anyone else may be doing. Eating occurs in one room in the house, with a regular table setting. The relative rigidity of this environmental control removes the overeater from uncertainty, and emphasizes the need to remain aware of what and how much is being eaten.

Reading a book or a newspaper or watching TV at the chosen eating place is also interdicted since there is the problem of subordinating the eating activity within another context that masks the food input. Once balanced eating habits are established, the need for such constraints should substantially diminish.

The social environment in which eating occurs is also relevant to control. Where possible, the overeater is encouraged to eat with someone, not alone. The presence of a second person seems to support eating-control efforts, even though the other person may have no awareness of the overeater's state of mind. Also, the support of significant members of the overeater's family and associates can be most helpful in the program of controlled eating and weight management. On the other hand, a hostile and antagonistic significant person can create a formidable barrier for the development of controls over eating. When overeating has been associated with an atmosphere of tension and stress at the dining table, it is clear that control of eating behavior can be undermined. The overeater has to recognize the effects of the tense social atmosphere, acknowledge that overeating is an inappropriate means of resolving the tension, and look for new ways to deal with the problem. Finally, good social support can be provided by such groups as Take Off Pounds Sensibly (TOPS), Weight Watchers, and Overeaters Anonymous.

Hypnotherapy offers the client the opportunity to explore, in a protected environment, the personal acceptability and feasibility of any proposed environmental change. The client can use the trance to vividly experience the new setting through active mental imagery for the purpose of checking out his or her reaction to the change. It can also be used to reinforce the effectiveness of a change that has been found useful, or to explore ways in which to make a desired change feasible. As in so many psychotherapeutic strategies useful with the overeater, the well-kept NICE diary remains a key to important leads for the planning and development of environmental controls.

The Strategy of Self-Reward

The psychotherapeutic strategy of self-reward is particularly relevant for the overeater who is committed to the goal of becoming a balanced eater. Typically, the uncontrolled eater has had a background replete with recriminations, impingements upon self-esteem, and barbs of social devaluation because of nonconformity to the physical standards of the group.

In contrast, the smoker generally has had a very different kind of exposure to social pressures. Even though recent institutional restrictions may designate separate areas for smokers and nonsmokers, the issue of social stigma is much less germane. The smoker does not continuously present a physical marker of variance from the body norm to his or her group. To be sure, the smoker who has had previous unsuccessful efforts at becoming a nonsmoker may experience doubts about the self, with concomitant feelings of helplessness and even hopelessness that impinge upon the self-concept, but there is no overload of general social criticism to endanger the smoker's self-esteem further. The uncontrolled eater, however, experiences repeated social condemnation. Thus, the strategy of self-reward not only sustains motivation for acquiring balanced eating but also helps to build or restore the person's self-esteem as part of the broader therapeutic outcome.

The details of the strategy of self-reward are set forth in Chapter 11 with respect to the smoker, and they apply to the uncontrolled eater as well. The central principle is that there should be ample opportunities for the individual to celebrate achievement. Thus, the unit of time for accomplishment to be noted should be sufficiently short so that a sense of achievement can be experienced on a daily basis or even more frequently. Each successful demonstration merits endorsement by the client, and by a social support network as well. It must be remembered that the new step has occurred in spite of the counteracting force of hundreds of repetitions of the older uncontrolled eating behavior. The unit of success should not be permitted to slip by unnoticed. As the client progresses in the program, and the occasions for self-reward are experienced again and again, the level of aspiration for what constitutes accomplishment may rise in terms of scope and complexity, building upon strengthened self-esteem and the goals that have been achieved in the control of eating. However, the basic principle should be kept in mind that the self-rewards *must* remain frequent and meaningful. Most overeaters have a long way to go before they can catch up with peers in regard to their body image, and uncertainties remain even in the face of obvious objective evidence of accomplishments.

The client is encouraged to plan self-rewards to be used as earned. Eating of tempting foods may sometimes be permitted or necessary in the total management of a program, but such an activity should be reserved for a special occasion such as a date, a celebration, and so forth, and not planned as a reward.

An end-of-the-day period of time set aside for endorsing the self is a valuable part of the self-reward strategy. The client is encouraged to plan for a 10- to 15-minute quiet time period to relax deeply in trance and visualize each instance in the day when he or she was able to manage controlled eating. As these occurrences multiply and progress is recognized, the retrospective imagery may include a wider time span. On occasion, the client may fantasize about his or her appearance and functioning in the not-too-distant future when the goals of the particular phase of learning to become a balanced eater have been met.

The psychotherapist and the client can learn to use hypnosis to endorse and amplify each of the strategies supporting the client's movement toward becoming a balanced eater and a manager of his or her own weight status. The therapist must continually remember, however, that it is the client who has the basic responsibility for learning ways of controlling eating and making use of these new skills, and that it is the client who has the right to make decisions about his or her own eating behavior. The therapist is a teacher, guide, knowledge resource, and trainer. The client is comanager of the treatment program and responsible for his or her own decisions. If progress is rapid or slow or even retrogressive, the role of the therapist is that of helping to solve problems and providing support, not that of acting as a moral judge. As cotherapists, the client and therapist have different responsibilities in the joint undertaking, but they share the goal of having the client achieve new eating habits that will make balanced eating an integral part of a way of life.

Overcoming Sexual Difficulties

EVOLUTIONARY AND SOCIETAL INFLUENCES

The biological, psychological, and social processes that have evolved over the millenia of human existence have established their effectiveness for reproductive sexuality. There can be more than reasonable assurance that reproduction of the human species will continue unless some human-initiated disaster, such as nuclear or chemical pollution, alters the genetic script.

The human sexual experience, however, extends beyond its essential reproductive function. Somewhere along the evolutionary path, humans became different in their sexual behavior from other mammals. They became independent of the "estrous clock" as a determiner of coital behavior, and body anatomy evolved to facilitate face-to-face sexual intercourse and social interaction. It is probable that some natural-selection factors operated that favored the survival of those human predecessors who experienced just a bit more sensual and interpersonal pleasure from sexual intercourse than other humans. For such couplings, the sexual behavior may have resulted in a bit more stable interpersonal bonding, which, in turn, may have fostered greater interdependence and cooperation that improved the survival potential of their offspring. One can surmise that, when the presence of a mature ovum in the Fallopian tube no longer was a necessary prerequisite for coitus, other factors became operative in the determination of human sexual behavior.

As it has evolved, human sexuality may be conceptualized as a compound need system, composed of both a biological aspect (e.g., neurohumoral, endocrine, sensory) and a psychosocial aspect. As a partial biological-need system, the sexual system shares some of the characteristics of other biological systems, such as those involving the need for food and water, in that consummatory activities discharge biological tension until there is a recurrence of the need state. When the tension level of the unfilled need becomes sufficiently high, it tends to dominate the behavioral field.

However, there are important differences between the biological character of the sexual-need system and the need systems that involve survival: Individual biological survival is *not* dependent upon the discharge of tension in the sexual-need system, even when tension levels are high. Regeneration of sexual tension does not follow the regular, cyclical patterns of the other survival-need systems. Tension in the sexual-need system is usually experienced as a positive state of arousal, in contrast to, for example, the survival needs of hunger and thirst. Finally, sexual activity that may have been capable of discharging sexual tension may undergo a valence shift from being highly positive to being neutral or even negative.

The psychosocial component of the sexual-need system has become much more important as a determinant of sexuality than the biological component, especially as the individual matures. The psychosocial component is determined by cultural–developmental learning, as well as by forces in the person's immediate life space. The variability in both the biological and the psychosocial components of human sexuality insures large individual differences in the degree to which the sexual-need system occupies a central position in the person's life. It also insures large individual differences in the character of sexual needs. For some individuals, sexual gratification depends more or less exclusively on genital release of sexual tension. For others, sexual satisfaction requires a broad range of erogenous experiences within a caring relationship. In some cases, orgasmic release is not of central importance. However, when such an important area of the human experience as sexual activity lacks or loses its pleasurable value, or acquires a negative character, then there is a strong possibility that the disruption of sexual behavior reflects difficulties involving aspects of the person's life that go beyond the biological sphere.

Both the reproductive and nonreproductive aspects of human sexuality undoubtedly affected (and were affected by) the social interactions and the social organization of humans, leading to customs and regulations of sexual behavior in all societies. What is striking is the great diversity of these customs and regulations that evolved as different cultures, isolated as they were from each other, defined the many facets of human sexuality within their own historical experience. The potential for stress associated with sexuality also increased as sexual behavior became embedded in the "dos and don'ts" of society.

Since World War I, there has been an accelerating pace of change in the social attitudes and expectations concerning the human sexual experience in the United States and other Western countries. Changes in sexual behavior seem to be closely related to the economic, political, and technological–industrial changes that were set in motion by two World Wars and a severe depression. Industrial expansion, transportation mobility, population movements, and women's suffrage not only influenced broad aspects of cultural expectations in general, but also had a major bearing on interpersonal relationships.

Two sets of factors, however, seem to have been especially significant in regard to their impact on sexual attitudes, expectations, and behaviors. First, and highly important, were the changes in the economic, educational, political, and legal status of women. Although many women had worked outside the home, it was not until World War I that a major mobilization of women into the work force took place. Then, immediately after the war, women made a significant advance toward equal citizenship with the acquisition of voting rights. An even more massive expansion of women in the out-of-home work force occurred during World War II. This time women did not return to work in the home only, and currently almost all women experience some degree of economic independence as part of their lives. Education beyond elementary school, vocational training, work mobility, and life with some degree of economic independence have become expectations of both sexes.

The new economic power of women brought significant changes in the family. In many instances the woman needed or wanted to work outside the home. This involved social and vocational contacts with men other than her spouse or partner. It also became a statement of her capacity to maintain herself by her own efforts if it ever became necessary (even though many single women, especially those with children, are impoverished). Working outside the home was an important step toward greater parity with respect to many aspects of the marital relationship, including the sexual.

Important questions arise concerning the long-term effects on sexual behavior of this economic reorientation between the sexes. There are clear indications that the traditional patterns of sexual behavior were powerfully determined by women's economic dependency on men. Thus, the guidelines for sexual behavior that developed in that context are viewed with both suspicion and uncertainty in regard to their relevance in the new economic circumstances. Women, as well as men, are asking whether the sexual experiences of women can or should be comparable to those of men. Can the traditional regulation of sexual behavior be set aside without threatening marriage or a committed partnership? How do the partners in a sexual relationship deal with changed expectations when they are still deeply immersed in a society where older traditions remain strong?

Uncertainty, conflict, and heightened stress are inevitable in any society experiencing a transition from clearly defined modes of behavior (whether or not they were strictly observed) to alternatives whose short- and long-term values are yet to be determined. It is predictable that many individuals, given such indeterminancy, will experience distinctly heightened anxiety about their own sexual behavior, their own roles, and the reactions of their partners. It is not surprising, therefore, that an increasing number of individuals of both sexes are concerned about the adequacy of their sexual functioning. The new awareness of sexual problems and the broad acceptance of open and varied sexual behavior in the media have led to an increase of research on disturbances in male and female sexuality and of clinical treatment approaches.

The second important set of factors that has influenced sexual attitudes, expectations, and behaviors has been the ready availability of inexpensive and effective birth-control devices, together with the relatively low health risk associated with their use. The decreased fear of pregnancy has undoubtedly contributed to the freedom to explore the nonreproductive, recreational aspects of sex. This has been an important factor in the increased frequency with which sexually active men and women have sexual experiences with more than one partner. Not only may this contribute to the sexual enjoyment each partner may be able to give to the other, but it may also provide a comparative base for assessing a particular sexual experience. For many individuals, it does not matter what they or their partners actually say or do. The very awareness of the potential for evaluation can heighten stress. It can lead to feelings of sexual inadequacy and disturbed sexual functioning.

The psychosocial determinants of sexual behavior not only reflect the foregoing societal influences, but include all sorts of misconceptions and attitudes about sexuality and sexual activity as well. As described by Masters and Johnson,[1] the human sexual response may be divided into four phases: namely, excitement, plateau (maintaining excitement level), orgasm, and resolution (lowering of excitement).

---

1. W. Masters and V. Johnson. *Human Sexual Response*. Boston: Little, Brown, 1966.

The excitement and plateau phases of the sexual response are principally dependent upon the modification of the blood-flow pattern in the genital organs and in the pelvic area. Through neurohumoral activation, there is a change in the arteriovascular circulation from the hemodynamics of the resting state to a state where the inflow of blood to the genital organs exceeds the blood outflow. The special tissues of the genital organs become filled with blood, and the changes in valvular function maintain this "back-pressure" with a consequent erection of the penis and clitoris, transudation of the vaginal wall, and stretching of the genital tissues, leading to heightened sensory feedback to the individual. Continuous excitatory input is necessary for this hemodynamic pressure ratio to be maintained. Thus, any psychobiological factor that reduces the excitatory input or alters blood flow may lead to a loss of engorgement and sensory feedback. Stress and anxiety are prime factors that may lead to such a decrement in sexual arousal–excitatory levels.

The orgasmic phase of the sexual response entails muscle contraction, in contrast to the hemodynamic vascular phenomena of the excitement and plateau phases. Of course, for the contractions to occur there must exist tissues that are stretched and engorged with blood, a sensory feedback mechanism with an escalating level, a neurological pattern that permits organized rhythmical contractions, and a release or trip mechanism. The psychobiological-trigger mechanism is dependent on a complex of variable factors. Under some circumstances, the threshold for release may rise, requiring substantially higher excitatory levels for the tripping mechanism to function; under other circumstances, the threshold may be lowered. Once again, misconceptions, fears, and antipathies or resentments toward the partner may interfere with satisfactory orgasmic release.

The need for help in resolving sexual difficulties, and the techniques that have been developed in treatment, are all closely related to the psychosocial fabric that shapes and cloaks human sexuality.

HYPNOTIC TRANCE AND LOVE-MAKING PHENOMENA

It is noteworthy that some of the conditions that facilitate hypnotic trance are characteristic of aroused emotional states associated with pleasurable sexual functioning. This has long been known to poets and lovers. The English literature is replete with descriptions of "entranced states" experienced by sexual partners intimately absorbed in making love. Closed eyes, privacy, and secure surroundings are part of this scene.

The experience of hypnosis occurs most readily when the individual has limited his or her responsiveness to a very narrow range of sensory input from the environment, along with a heightened awareness of physical sensations. This heightened awareness of the physical self is facilitated by eye closure, which also enables the person to appreciate and respond more fully to inner emotional states, to roam more freely in imagination and fantasy, and to tolerate more comfortably the flow of internal events and experiences without the necessity for critical and defensive controls or inhibitions. A significant part of almost every induction procedure is the condition of trust and rapport developed between the person and the one who helps to guide the hypnotic experience, often a therapist. Although highly vigorous mental and physical experiences do occur during trance, the induction phase seems to be strongly facilitated by physical and psychological relaxation. This relaxation is supported by focusing attention upon some pleasurable or nonthreatening idea, object, or event. The emphasis by the guide on relaxing, letting things happen, and freeing oneself from demands that certain events must occur seems to facilitate movement into that state of consciousness called hypnosis.

How closely this description parallels the conditions conducive to a satisfying love experience! Sexual fulfillment is more likely to occur when the partners feel secure enough with each other to permit their individual vulnerabilities to be exposed without fear of being hurt— when "touch and glow" create an intimacy and union between two individuals, temporarily dissolving the separation and aloneness that is a typical part of the human condition. For the time being, the boundary zone that our individual skins inevitably re-establish is set aside.

GENERAL PSYCHOTHERAPEUTIC OBJECTIVES, STRATEGIES, AND THE USE OF HYPNOSIS

Sexual functioning depends on a complex interaction of anatomy, physiology, psychology, and the social environment, insofar as these can be meaningfully separated as factors. When a person has reached a point of distress over sexual functioning that impels him or her to search for help, it may be assumed that the source of distress arises from one or more of these interacting factors. There may be biochemical interference associated with alcohol, Thorazine, morphine, tranquilizers, or antihypertensive medications, for example. Or there may be disturbances of neurophysiological functioning associated with disability and illness, such as diabetes mellitus, spinal cord injury, or debilitating disease.

Although from the clinical perspective, the greatest proportion of sexual dysfunction is primarily associated with psychosocial determinants, an essential part of sex therapy is the assessment of the anatomical and physiological status of the individual, followed by such medical remediation as may be indicated. Medical intervention may involve minor alteration of medication; surgical intervention; the treatment of infection, trauma, and degenerative processes; major changes in the general metabolic state of the patient; and/or general health care. Yet, even when organic factors have been found to be an important component of the sexual disturbance, and even when medical remediation has been reasonably effective, psychological problems almost always remain to be dealt with, just as in the case of the sexually troubled person whose anatomy and physiology have been found to be free of any relevant problems.

The treatment program for the psychotherapy of sexual difficulties derives directly from an analysis of the nonreproductive aspects of human sexuality, with an emphasis on psychosocial factors. Since only the person has knowledge about himself or herself that enables the therapist to help in dealing with the sexual issues and problems, it is necessary for the client to assume an active role in therapy. That is why the concept of the client as cotherapist is so appropriate.

It makes a great deal of difference whether the presenting problem is more or less limited to the sexual sphere or whether it is only one manifestation of inadequacy in many life areas. Some individuals, for example, experience not only little pleasure with sex, but little pleasure in general. In such a case, the psychological problems are much broader than those in the sexual area, and the psychotherapeutic approach needs to be directed to these life difficulties before there can be an effective change in sexual functioning. In contrast is the individual whose loss of pleasure is limited to the sexual sphere. In this case, considerable value may be derived from psychotherapeutic interventions that are directly focused on current sexual functioning. However, what is often needed in addition is psychotherapeutic attention to both developmentally healthy and developmentally negative experiences that have become associated with sexuality.

There are many psychotherapeutic approaches to sex therapy; examples include behavior modification, desensitization, insight-oriented psychotherapy, and rational–emotive cognitive restructuring. No matter what the psychotherapeutic orientation is, however, hypnotic trance can be used to increase its effectiveness. Also, careful diagnostic differentiation of the nature of the disturbance is important in order for the therapist and client to more effectively plan an approach to remediation. Ultimately, the criteria of effective treatment include improved sexual functioning and increased satisfaction.

One other matter cannot be ignored, and that is the issue of responsible sexual activity. Sexual activity that does not consider the needs, feelings, and values of the partner is irresponsible. Furthermore, sexual activity that does not include adequate precautions against the possibility of unwanted pregnancy is also irresponsible.

The following sections elaborate a number of general considerations and guidelines that can be incorporated within a wide range of psychotherapeutic approaches.

Self-Acceptance as a Sexual Being

A major objective in the psychotherapy of the client with sexual problems is to help the person achieve a fuller acceptance of the self as a sexual being—as someone who is not always obliged to conform to other people's definition of or norms for sexual expression. It helps to recognize that sexual feelings and behavior vary widely in terms of type, frequency, intensity, and quality among people, and that genital sexuality and orgasmic release are not necessarily the sine qua non of the human sexual experience. It also helps to recognize that people change over time and to discover how one feels about one's own sexuality. The individual is then freer to change sexual behavior, if that is desired, while maintaining acceptance of his or her integrity as a sexual being.

Value Reorientation

Two sex-value frameworks seem to be especially coercive in inducing significant levels of psychological stress: the negativity framework and the power framework.

The negativity framework is the value orientation that associates sexual feelings, attitudes, and behavior with shame, guilt, devaluation, and exploitation. Its broad negativity suffuses an unhappy and uncomfortable aura onto everything associated with sexuality. For stress to be reduced, a shift needs to occur toward more positively oriented values that allow a view of sex as life-enhancing, creative, and emotionally satisfying.

The second value orientation, the power framework, relates sexual functioning to power, performance, and comparative achievement (i.e., one's sexual "prowess" is compared to that of someone else). It is a value framework that carries over from the wider society's emphasis on competitive performance and achievement. These values are transferred to the sexual sphere so that men and women have become burdened with rigid standards of performance and outcomes—with mechanical guidelines that have been heard, portrayed, or read somewhere—and they place these not only on themselves but on each other. The consequence is a heavy dose of anxiety, which interferes with relaxation and deflects attention from the pleasure of interpersonal sharing upon which sexual fulfillment, in many cases, rests.

Values replacing the negativity and power frameworks are as applicable to homosexual relationships as they are to heterosexual relationships. They are consonant with the precepts of a wide range of religions and fit a wide range of life styles. For stress to be moderated, the reorientation of values has to permit the giving and receiving of sensual pleasure and the freeing up of "performance" standards in a caring, responsive, and responsible relationship, without bookkeeping ledgers.

Communication, Desensitization, and Anxiety Reduction

Negative feelings about sexuality tend to induce a self-perpetuating cycle whose effects become more and more capable of disrupting competent and satisfying sexual functioning. Sustained anxiety and apprehension create psychophysiological antagonists that disrupt the human sexual response. Furthermore, there is a strong tendency for repeated reactions of apprehension to become autonomous; that is, anxiety may be triggered independently of the circumstances originally associated with its evocation. The amelioration of anxiety, therefore, becomes a sine qua non, a precondition, for any significant psychotherapeutic movement toward satisfying sexual relations.

Intense shame, guilt, and anxiety about sexuality in general or about one's own sexual functioning generate avoidance and aversive behaviors that further isolate the individual from the possibility of pleasant, satisfying sexual experiences. Also, the individual is likely to avoid discussing sexual concerns with others and to resist exploring the origins of the negative feelings in himself or herself. Instead, sexual matters may be regarded as unimportant in one's life and devalued, or projected outward as antisex rhetoric. When a person finally does seek outside help, it usually indicates that the problems associated with sex have become more stressful than the prospect of discussing sexual matters. It also suggests that self-help efforts have not been successful.

Because the client has to describe the nature of his or her sexual difficulties even in the presence of uncomfortable feelings, and because the therapist is able to facilitate the communication, the client begins to feel less threatened by matters that previously were taboo. In this way, the diagnostic requirements of the therapeutic relationship contribute to the desensitization process so important in the working through of sexual problems. The therapist eases communication by using the client's sex language or, when needed, by providing terminology that clearly identifies a body part or sex function. The client comes to appreciate that a sexual problem merits the same kind of therapeutic concern that is given to other life problems.

Topics covered in the exploration of the present difficulties include the earliest manifestations of the problems, whether change in function or satisfaction has occurred precipitously or over time, the partner's reaction to the problem, the client's expectation of the future course of the difficulty, and so forth. Attitudes, feelings, and gaps or errors in information become evident. The therapist serves not only as a source of information, but also as a source of encouragement when the client learns that similar sexual difficulties have been experienced by others who have managed to deal effectively with them.

Often it is a couple rather than just one individual who is involved in sex therapy. The assessment sessions may be the first time that either partner has ever heard the other partner speak openly about sexual concerns, desires, needs, problems, or issues. When the partners have been alone with each other, this important area of discourse may not have seemed available to them because of fear of what might be revealed. In the security of the psychotherapeutic setting, however, where a professional helper is available to keep distress within safe limits, the airing and sharing of problems become possible.

Hypnotherapeutic interventions can be most helpful in the communication and desensitization phases of the treatment program. To clients who have difficulty talking about their sexual problems, the hypnotic trance can be described as a special state of consciousness that will enable them to be relatively calm and detached even while discussing emotionally stressful concerns. Also, clients should be encouraged with the assurance that they can develop skill in utilizing hypnosis to facilitate coping with their problems.

Sometimes a client needs time to adjust to the content and feelings that have just been disclosed during trance. In such cases, the client can be encouraged to develop a temporary amnesia for these materials until such time as he or she feels better able to cope with the situation. When posthypnotic amnesia is not readily available to the client, the stressful content may be repetitively reviewed while in trance, with the suggestion that with each review the client will feel a lowering of the level of stress and an increased confidence in being able to cope with the situation.

The client's sense of control over events during the course of therapy can be emphasized by the use of the Chevreul pendulum (see Chapter 2, pp. 29–31) to obtain permission for any hypnotherapeutic exploration. The "inner part of the mind" becomes part of the dialogue between client and therapist to regulate the pace, direction, and character of the coping efforts. Affirmative consent also emphasizes the cotherapist role of the client.

As a cotherapist, it is important that the client learn how to relax readily and extensively, induce autohypnosis, utilize imagery and fantasy in all phases of therapy, make use of posthypnotic amnesia, and practice positive self-suggestions. Even for clients who are readily able to communicate about their sexual problems, the hypnotic trance can be useful in facilitating recall of previously effective sexual functioning, exploring the circumstances surrounding the onset of present difficulties, increasing awareness of conditions that trigger anxiety in the sexual realm, examining events that may be indirectly related to the sexual problem, and reducing tension when engaged in rehabilitative sexual behavior.

In couples therapy, both partners may make use of the trance state as a means for easing tension while discussing sexual problems together. If psychodrama techniques are used for the purpose of exchanging roles between the partners, the trance state during the role play seems to give permission for each partner to portray the other's behavior more emphatically. This makes it easier to clarify the sexual messages that have been conveyed between them. Thus, the hypnotic-trance state not only is useful for assessing sexual difficulties, but also is an important therapeutic medium for various phases of the psychotherapy program.

Sexual Awareness and Integrity

Typically, the disruption of responsive and healthy sexual functioning results from some kind of psychological barrier. The inhibitory forces may be a consequence of disquieting attitudes about one's body derived from religious precepts, social-class attitudes, misinformation, myths, or parental models; or there may be a complex of negative feelings about the meaning and consequences of sexual behavior; or deeply frightening beliefs may be held about the psychological effects of certain autoerotic sexual acts; or life experiences may have sexually traumatized an individual.

Psychotherapeutic strategies for restoring the integrity of sexual functioning have two broad goals. The first of these is the need to identify the disruptive ideas, feelings, and experiences related to the dysfunction, with a view to developing wholeness as a sexual being. The second goal is the restoration of optimal functioning compatible with the individual's values and situation.

The goal of identifying dysfunctional sexual attitudes and experiences is well served by a comprehensive sex history, a review of sex knowledge, and a survey of sex attitudes. The re-education process makes use of discussion, reading, and audiovisual presentations to give the client more adequate knowledge about the male and female bodies, especially in those areas where lack of knowledge or misinformation has been found to exist. These presentations also contribute to the desensitization and freeing of communication about sexual matters. Restructuring of sexual attitudes is facilitated by the nature of the client–therapist interactions, of course, but it can also benefit from the sharing of views and experiences with other people in a therapeutic setting that includes films, tapes, and group discussion. Sexual awareness and fulfillment are drastically constricted when the major concern is limited to the genital area and orgasmic response. It is important to appreciate that eroticization of large areas of skin not only enhances the specific pleasure of genital union but also expands the capacity for intimacy and interpersonal contact between the partners. The expansion of sexual awareness includes learning about alternative modes of sexual arousal, sensual pleasuring, and sexual satisfaction. It includes new ways of perceiving sexual-behavior options, including the awareness of genital and extragenital sexuality and the importance of interpersonal interaction. It includes awareness of sexual behaviors that others have found enjoyable and meaningful. The consciousness of alternatives at least provides the individual with a choice as to whether or not these options fit the individual's own and his or her partner's needs and values. It makes possible the recognition that sexual behavior can be a changing, evolving, personal, and interpersonal experience.

Should there be a decision to explore alternative sexual behaviors, learning occurs in a therapeutic context where support is available. The expansion of the spectrum of possible ways of sexual experiencing tends to facilitate the growth of the person's capacity for sharing, communication, and intimacy with his or her partner. The enlarged life space seems to reduce significantly the psychological stress associated with a narrow view of human sexuality.

The restoring of sexual integrity often involves the client in *in vivo* sexual experiences. The rehabilitation experiences may be designed to broaden the client's appreciation of the scope of sexuality, to give the client a greater awareness of his or her own sexual needs and behavior, or to provide the client with special sexual techniques that have value for a particular sexual difficulty. An example of the latter is the method in which circumcoronal pressure beneath the glans of the erect penis by a cooperating partner helps the male to re-educate the ejaculatory impulse. To improve the female's capability for experiencing vaginal sensations and active participation during coitus, the Kegel pubococcygeus muscle exercises are recommended.[2] These exercises consist of tightening and relaxing the anogenital muscles. Still another example of a specific intervention that becomes part of the wholeness and integrity of sexual functioning is instruction in alterna-

---

2. A. H. Kegel. Sexual Functions of the Pubococcygeus Muscle. *Western Journal of Obstetrics and Gynocology*, 1952, Vol. 60, 521–524.

tive coital positions to enable the couple to circumvent certain physical problems.

Masters and Johnson[3] introduced the sensate-focus, graduated exercises as a method whereby a couple can explore sensual pleasuring and sexual arousal independently of the demand to perform coitally. These nondemand sensual interactions emphasize verbal and nonverbal communication between the partners. They guide the client in how both to receive and to give sensual pleasure. Each new exercise has a progressively stronger potential for sexual arousal along with sensory pleasuring. The client becomes aware of any part of the body that is responsive to sensory stimulation. There is a growing awareness of the broader range of body sensations that may take on sexual connotations; it becomes clear that sexuality is not limited to direct genital contact. Of crucial importance in the sensate-focus exercises is encouraging each partner to let the other know what pleases and what does not please, to guide the partner verbally and manually in doing what is sensually and sexually pleasurable, and to change any particular aspect at any point where it seems to lose its pleasurable character. The goal for both partners is to please each other and to be pleased, not to give a sexual performance or to "prove" sexual competence. In the intimate atmosphere created by the partners for themselves, mutual support, sharing, communication, and awareness of each other's sexuality are fostered.

Clients who are anxious about the sensate-focus experience are encouraged to induce trance in themselves to lower the general tension level. They are encouraged to continue reminding themselves that they will feel more and more relaxed as the exercises proceed. As distracting thoughts and stimuli become screened out, the trance state further enhances awareness of pleasurable sensations. Each partner is asked to engage in the self-suggestion that his or her entire being will focus upon each new awareness coming from his or her own body and from the nearness of the partner, and that for the duration of the exercise the trance state will help the partners to set aside the world outside.

In the sensate-focus exercises, the partners alternate between more active and more passive roles in sensual pleasuring and being pleasured. When a client is being pleasured, the self-suggestion is made that each pleasurable contact by the partner, each touch, each

3. W. Masters and V. Johnson. *Human Sexual Inadequacy.* Boston: Little, Brown, 1970.

communication will become enriched by the client's own increased sensitivity and greater receptivity to the partner. Each participant is encouraged to become especially aware of the closeness of the partner, their sharing of the experience, and the feelings of intimacy arising out of the new freedom to talk openly about their sensual and sexual desires. In the later phases of the sensate-focus exercises, the trance suggestions focus upon heightened receptivity to sexual communications from the partner and from the individual's own arousal. The readiness to guide, communicate, and recognize the sensual-sexual responses as a willingly experienced part of the self engages the therapeutic process of restoring sexual integrity.

Some sexual problems, such as anhedonia and anorgasmia, are sometimes more readily overcome when the client begins the relearning process by discovering his or her own body responsiveness apart from a sexual partner. The self-pleasuring, autoerotic sexual situation makes this possible. A private environment selected by the client that is relatively free of tension and distraction is essential. It is also necessary that the client have complete control over the manner of his or her own sexual expression and be accountable only to the self. Self-pleasuring is presented in therapy as one possible way to facilitate sexual functioning and fulfillment.

Not infrequently, however, the same factors that have contributed to the disruption of sexual function also make self-pleasuring either taboo, anxiety-arousing, or of uncertain access. Self-pleasuring (masturbation) has a long history of social disapproval and religious condemnation. The historical necessities for tribal and species survival generated mechanisms of social control that not only have long outlived their intended purpose, but have been a source of continual anxiety, shame, and guilt right into the present day. Thus, the demythologizing of self-pleasuring and its perception as a normal, healthy sexual option for women and men is frequently a first step in the psychotherapeutic strategy.

An almost invariable question is why the term "self-pleasuring" rather than "masturbation" is used. It can be explained how a perfectly good term, such as "masturbation," can acquire such negative social and emotional connotations that what could be a potentially healthy experience is canceled out by the fear and mythology surrounding the word.

Presentation of the contemporary view of self-pleasuring, the use of bibliotherapy, and the shared viewing of films of individuals of the same and the other sex demonstrating self-pleasuring methods are all indicated. In discussing the films, the client is given ample opportunity to raise questions and explore any antipathies that even the term "masturbation" evokes, until not only has desensitization occurred, but a positive anticipation of the potential for sexual reeducation is recognized. The films and the discussion bring in the possibility of the use of a vibrator, but this may be of value only to those clients who accept it comfortably. When the client indicates a readiness to engage in autoerotic experiences, it is worthwhile to make use of ideometer signaling as a means of exploring whether the "inner part of the mind" is comfortable with the decision.

The client is encouraged to make use of hypnotic trance to heighten sensory, sexual, and pleasurable awareness of each aspect of his or her own self-pleasuring. The initial "trance detachment" often helps the client to lower the anxiety level, to exclude external distractions, and to become disinhibited to the flux of sexual feeling. The principal goal is to have the client experience sexual arousal, to permit the arousal to build to a peak, and for orgasmic release to occur in a context of pleasure, free of performance demands. When this stage has been achieved, the client is encouraged to use hypnotic trance to activate vivid interpersonal sexual imagery during self-pleasuring. Finally, for most clients, the experience of sexual gratification by oneself is then transposed to the interpersonal sphere where new learnings, shared with the partner, become integrated into the total range of sexual expression of the couple. The trance state can continue to be used as a means of freeing communication and maintaining reduced stress levels.

Security Enhancement: Example of Activating Positive Sexual Experiences

The feeling of security can be conceptualized as a network of complex cognitions and affects that permits an individual to make decisions about action and commitment, even though uncertainty and a certain amount of risk remain. The feeling of security is more than the absence of an imminent threat to one's well-being, although such an awareness is an important component of the security experience. The security complex includes such determinants as (1) awareness of some degree of control over one's situation; (2) ability to predict, even if only for the immediate future, how one's body will function and the general characteristics of the environments in which one will have to function; (3) awareness of the extent of one's ability to mobilize reasonably adequate coping skills if a problem should emerge; and (4) readiness to expand one's life space if the desire or a special occasion should arise. The enhancement of the feeling of security may involve the strengthening of any one or more of the determinants of the cognitive–affective complex. The growth of security in the sphere of sexual functioning helps the client to risk exploring alternative ways of sexual functioning in order to develop more adequate and satisfying sexual relations.

Hypnotherapeutic experiences can be used to facilitate any psychotherapeutic strategy directed toward the enhancement of the individual's feelings of security. The use of the trance state for relaxation and interruption of stress escalation has already been described in earlier chapters. Skill in reducing tension and modifying anxiety expands the individual's feeling of control over his or her own destiny. The hypnotic state is also available as a facilitating medium to explore cognitions and feelings about specific conditions that precipitate sexual stress, as well as the options that may be available to modify these conditions. The client can apply the learned tension-reducing skills during sexual activity to enhance the sensual pleasures deriving from awareness of his or her own body sensations, while also becoming more sensitively tuned in to the partner's verbal and nonverbal communications.

The following discussion of erectile difficulty during the excitement and plateau phases of the sexual response serves to illustrate the use of hypnosis in activating hope and enhancing security. When there have been several or repeated experiences with erectile inadequacy, a man may come to a new sexual encounter with considerable anxiety about his sexual response. The expectation that he will once again experience erectile problems and be unable to function "normally" may concentrate his attention on performance rather than on experiencing sensual pleasure. The anxiety and doubt interfere with the excitatory process by decreasing awareness of the full range of sensory feedback from the erogenous areas of the body, and by diverting attention to the threatening images of still another unsatisfying sexual encounter.

The activation of hope for more satisfying sexual functioning can serve as a most useful therapeutic intervention in helping such a client to shift from negative expectations toward a mindset that permits the arousal–excitement phase to develop. For a client who has had a previous history of satisfactory arousal experiences, hypnotic trance can be used to activate the person's memories of them, to renew awareness of the feelings of full sexual arousal and excitement with lowered anxiety, and to reassimilate that functioning into the image of himself as a sexual person. The hypnotic trance becomes a medium for intensifying the vividness of the experiences and for granting permission to renew these satisfying experiences as an integral part of the self.

The client in the following example was a 38-year-old married man with two children. His relationship with his wife was positive and stable. The erectile difficulties were of four years' duration and had become more frequent as time went by. There had been four previous sessions (two conjoint with his wife) with training in the use of hypnotic trance.

THERAPIST: You indicated that it was all right for you to go back to a time when you clearly remember having a very satisfying sexual experience . . . where there was full and exciting arousal and participation on your part . . . When you are back into that time and place . . . signal by raising your right index finger. . . . [The client's right index finger rises after about thirty seconds' delay.]

Very good . . . Now go deeply into your own inner space . . . Everything of the present is closed off except your connection with myself here if there should be need of contact . . . Re-experience the full and satisfying sexual response of your body in that sexual encounter with your partner . . . Let yourself be totally enclosed in that experience . . . You may need five minutes of world time, but your experience time may last as long as needed . . . Signal with your index finger when the experience is finished. . . .

[There is a slight smile on the client's face, and limited body movement. After about five minutes, he sighs deeply; then his index finger rises.]

T: You may or may not feel like sharing this experience with me at this moment . . . Give yourself time to fully absorb the satisfying parts of the sexual experience . . . Note how involved you were, how your thoughts and sensitivities were in the situation, not diverted elsewhere . . . how your body responded without special pressures

. . . Would you like to go back and relive this satisfying sexual encounter once more? [The client signals "yes" with his right index finger.] Be even more fully aware of how naturally and fully your body responds . . . If you choose, you can experience what is happening as if it were happening in the present . . . Signal when you are finished. . . .

A client may be guided through the same experience several times, or may relive other satisfying sexual encounters in the past, before an inquiry is made into these past memories. The following discussion with the client described above took place following the trance experience—that is, during the waking state of consciousness:

THERAPIST: What was especially pleasing about these relived experiences?

CLIENT: I think what was really great was that I could feel myself becoming erect and staying erect throughout the whole experience. I felt really pleased with myself and almost began to think that if it could happen so easily in the past, why couldn't it be part of me once more? The last time through, I really became aware of some positive sensations and liked it.

T: As you can see, all the components of a full and satisfying sexual experience are stored in you; they are part of your mind and your body. Your body knows the way, once the interferences are removed. How could it have been better?

C: I'd be satisfied to settle for just the way it was. If it could only begin happening right now, regularly. You know . . . I was concentrated on what was happening in me and my wife seemed to disappear. I would like to have good erection but want to stay connected to my wife. . . .

T: Why not? If that's an important part of your full sexual satisfaction, that's how it will be. She'll be more in it as your security in your own body reaction grows. . . .

[At this point, the therapist invites the client to enter the trance state once again:] Would you give yourself the cue to go more fully into the trance state . . . and then take off for a trip into the future . . . perhaps days, weeks, or even longer. See yourself enjoying a fully satisfying sexual encounter with your wife. Let yourself enjoy the experience . . . Signal with your fingers when you are ready to talk with me. . . .

C: [A few minutes go by; the client then sighs and raises his index finger.] That was beautiful.

T: What was the date?

C: Gee, I didn't notice. It seemed to me that it was only a month or so off, but I'm not sure.

T: Part of you is already anticipating a time in the relatively near future. Remember, that is not a demand on you . . . but your inner feeling that things should move along reasonably well. . . .

The hypnotic trance continued to be used to intensify the imagery of satisfying sexual functioning and to encourage anticipation of such repeated occurrences in the future.

Relationship Growth: Example of Uncovering Interpersonal Stress

Difficulties in the general relationship of the partners may create stress in the sexual sphere as well as vice versa. Feelings of frustration, anger, resentment, and rejection stemming from conflicts over money, personal habits, and other aspects of the relationship may find their way into the bedroom as a covert, hidden agenda that disturbs sexual functioning. So long as this covert agenda persists, psychotherapeutic efforts must be directed at dealing with these conflicts and related conditions rather than with the sexual problems alone. When the covert agenda has been removed from the area of sexual functioning, the probability of a satisfactory resolution of the sexual difficulties is substantially increased. This is especially true in cases where the fullness of sexual satisfaction rests on the shared intimacy, affirmation, and affection between the sexual partners.

Many approaches in sex therapy are quite dependent upon a warm and caring relationship between the partners. The partners are encouraged to talk to each other about their sexual desires, preferences, and distastes. The partners often have to learn both verbal and nonverbal ways of expressing affection and sexual intimacy that are acceptable to each other. When mind reading has been set aside in favor of direct sharing with each other, then a major step toward better sexual functioning has been taken. With freer communication, it is easier for the partners to learn more responsive ways to express intimacy as a sexual couple and to recognize the potential for change in sexual expression as the relationship evolves.

Hypnosis can be helpful in uncovering the earliest manifestations of problems in sex functioning, with a view to improving misunderstandings and conflicts in the sexual and nonsexual aspects of the relationships. The example below is that of a 48-year-old man who became aware of erectile problems in the last two of his six years of marriage to his second wife. He had not experienced difficulty in erectile functioning during his first marriage despite much quarreling. Prior to the following trance excerpt, there had been six psychotherapy sessions, part of which were devoted to training in the use of hypnotic trance.

THERAPIST: [After asking the client to go back in time, the therapist continues:] And when you have reached the time when you first experienced any problems in achieving or maintaining a full erection, signal with your right index finger. [After about two to three minutes, the client's index finger rises.]

Let's check with the inner part of your mind if it is okay for you to relive this experience so that you can learn how to function with more satisfaction sexually in the present. [Again, the right index finger, the "yes" finger, goes up.]

Okay. Observe yourself going through that experience, especially taking note of any disharmonious, stressful aspects of the experience, and signal when you are finished. [The client's index finger rises after about four minutes.] Is it all right for you to share, in detail, everything that happened?

CLIENT: I guess that I first felt something when we were in the living room that evening. Marianne seemed distant and distracted, even before we started up to bed. She was reading, and when I spoke to her it was treated more like an interruption. When we got upstairs, I got into bed first and turned on the little radio on the headboard. This had been a kind of signal we used when we wanted to let each other know that it would be nice to have sex that night. She got into bed and then got out again and went into the bathroom. She must have spent an awfully long time there because I found myself almost drifting off to sleep . . . Then, when she came back, sex didn't go right.

The course of therapy explored the circumstances associated with this earliest remembered experience of erectile dysfunction; special attention was given to concurrent feelings of malaise, resentment, and tension that might have been antagonistic to the flow of arousal. In the next few sessions, the wife joined the discussion of the couple's difficulties in their broader relationship. She too harbored resentments that were "aired and pared" as misunderstandings were cleared up and new ways of communicating with each other in both the sexual and nonsexual areas were practiced. Using autohypnosis, the husband also practiced transforming the first recalled experience of erectile difficulty into a fantasy in which everything went well and in which the factors that had interfered with sexual functioning were handled in such a way that they no longer blocked the sexual response.

Psychodrama can also be used to enrich the relationship between partners in nonsexual as well as sexual areas. Here again, the use of hypnotic trance is therapeutically advantageous. Partners seem to feel better able to function as protagonists, to experience their own and each other's roles more deeply, when they make use of the trance state while engaged in the psychodrama. The use of psychodrama for exploration of problems in the sexual sphere permits "role reversals" between the partners so that each can communicate his or her perception of how the other partner functions in addition to portraying his or her own behavior. Discussion of the differences validates the fundamental importance of the following principle: Unwarranted inferences about the other partner often become a source of misunderstanding when open communication could provide a basis for resolving difficulties. The psychodrama experience also influences the readiness of the partners to perceive sexuality as being more than genitality; to risk exploring alternate ways of relating to each other sexually; and to accept each other's sexuality as capable of change, as an evolving part of their total relationship.

The use of hypnosis in the psychotherapy of sexual dysfunction has such a high potential because of the significant role that abatement of fear and anxiety plays. Hypnosis is particularly useful in helping the client create a situation of relaxation and security to facilitate the uncovering of significant memories, the engagement in useful fantasy, and the focusing of attention on bodily sensations during the sensate-focus and self-pleasuring experiences. The objective is to reorient sexuality away from "performance achievement" and toward responsive and responsible satisfaction. Where life problems and conflicts interfere with sexual fulfillment, the trance state of consciousness can be incorporated within the psychotherapeutic process to facilitate their resolution.

Meeting the Challenge of
Sleep Disturbances

Sleep is a significant part of our life journey, occupying as it does about one-third of the human lifetime. The rhythms of awake activity and quiet rest are already manifested by the movement of the fetus as early as the midperiod of pregnancy, and the cycle of awake–rest continues until the final quietness of death ends all biorhythms.

Our human genetic structure has become encoded and programmed with many biorhythms as a response to eons of stimulation by and adaptation to the geophysical cycles of our planet: the cycles of light and dark, hot and cold, dry and wet, lunar gravitational pull, and many other recurrent cycles of physical influence. Cycles that recur at approximately 24-hour intervals are referred to as "circadian." Those that recur more frequently are referred to as "ultradian." In the adult, the cycle of awake–rest tends to be a circadian cycle. Since sleep consists of a number of stages including dreaming that cycle through the night, the sleep–dream cycle is designated an ultradian cycle.

From the evolutionary perspective, it is reasonable to hypothesize that the awake–rest cycle and the sleep–dream cycle must have had some adaptive function to have come into being and to have persisted into the present. It is clear that sleep deprivation for even relatively short periods of time leads the vast majority of people to experience a disturbance of their sense of well-being.

THE AWAKE–REST CYCLE

The sleep phase of the awake–rest cycle differs impressively among different species of mammals. The domesticated cow, for example, has a sleep phase of less than one hour out of the 24-hour period, whereas the opossum has a sleep phase of over 19 hours for the same period. The adult human's sleep phase is about seven to eight hours.

It is much easier to understand the adaptive-survival values of the wakeful part of the cycle than the sleep phase. There is a clear necessity for the organism to be awake and prepared to deal with environmental conditions in order to obtain food, mate for reproduction, and protect itself from predators. However, the dramatic change in the central nervous system during sleep, where there is paralysis of motor function, decreased awareness of external stimuli, and a great vulnerability to attack by predators, is more difficult to grasp from an adaptive-survival hypothesis. It is true that sleep in humans often follows sexual activity, which probably enhances the possibilities of fertilization. Also, digestion of food can occur more readily, and probably muscle tissue is restored with rest. It is clear that the factor of vulnerability to predators, threatening though it may seem to be for survival, has been a much less important factor than the adaptive-survival value of other aspects of sleep, for the fact remains that humans and other mammals have survived with this sleep stage, and continue to need to sleep.

THE SLEEP–DREAM CYCLE

In addition to the long circadian cycle of awake–rest, each mammalian species also has much shorter biorhythms that occur many times during the 24-hour period. These shorter biorhythms, of which the sleep-dream cycle is one, seem to be correlated with the brain size of the particular mammalian species. The elephant, with a brain size of 4600 grams, has a sleep–dream cycle of about 125 minutes; the adult human, with a brain size of 1320 grams, has a cycle of 95 minutes; the human infant, with a 460-gram brain size, has a 60-minute cycle; and the mouse, with a two-gram brain size, has a ten-minute cycle. Many physiological functions (e.g., hormonal secretions) go through a cycle of high and low intensity during the time period characteristic for that species. The sleep-dream cycle is such a 90- to 100-minute ultradian cycle in humans and is observable at some point in the awake–rest cycle when the rest phase reaches a certain level of ascendancy.

A rational therapeutic approach to the diagnosis and treatment of difficulties with sleep necessitates an awareness of (1) the neurophysiology of the circadian awake–rest and the ultradian sleep–dream cycles, and (2) the psychological factors and environmental influences that may disturb an individual's normal sleep pattern.

THE PHASES AND STAGES OF SLEEP

A number of discoveries and technological advances led to the establishment of sleep laboratories and renewed interest in the scientific
study of sleep and dreaming in the 1950s. The report that quiet sleep
could be distinguished from episodes in which the movement of the
eyes became much more active aroused interest in the possibility that
rapid eye movements (REM), being more like the scanning movements of wakefulness than the rolling eye movements of drowsiness,
might be correlated with dreaming. This conjecture has been amply
verified in the intervening years. There was also the possibility of
three types of polygraph recordings that could be used to measure
certain physiological events during sleep: recordings of brain waves
via the electroencephalogram (EEG), of muscle tonus via the electromyogram (EMG), and of eye movements via the electro-oculogram
(EOG).

The sleep–dream cycle is generally divided into two phases: (1) a
quiet phase, known as "non-REM (NREM) sleep" because there are
no rapid eye movements, any eye movement being slow and rare; and
(2) an active phase referred to as "REM sleep," manifested by vivid
dreaming and rapid eye movements.

Four stages have been identified, using EEG recordings, as defining depth of sleep. EEG changes in the successive stages of sleep are
marked by the gradual disappearance of alpha waves characteristic
of relaxed wakefulness, the appearance of "sleep spindles" in a sinu-
soidal wave pattern, and the appearance of "K-complex waves"
consisting of brief discharges of high voltage and slow waves. When
the slow waves occur 50% of the time, the sleeper has reached Stage
IV, the deepest stage of sleep. The person is most relaxed, with
relatively few body movements. It is most important to note that even
in the deepest stage of sleep, mental activity does not cease, although
it is poorly organized and the amount and clarity of any dreaming that
may occur are relatively limited.

Usually, the NREM and REM phases cycle every 90–100 minutes,
with REM appearing following the return to Stage I sleep. This occurs
three to six times during a typical night's sleep. The proportion of
time spent in REM sleep, however, increases in successive cycles.
REM may last only a few minutes during the first cycle, and as long as
60 minutes during the last. Also, as sleep progresses, there is a gradual

decrease of time spent in Stages III and IV, the deep-sleep stages of NREM sleep. The last two of the sleep–dream cycles of the night may lack Stages III and IV entirely.

The pattern of sleep also changes during the course of life. At birth, almost 50% of sleep time is spent in REM sleep. The older child's REM sleep is considerably shorter, about 25% of sleep time; during adult life, there is a further decrease to about 20%. The relatively large proportion of sleep time spent in Stages III and IV sleep by the older child decreases in the adult years, and in the senior years there may be little or no time spent in these deeper stages of sleep. Differences in the sleep–dream cycle patterns have relevance for the types of sleep disturbances that occur at different ages.

It is clear that sleep is not a period of suspended animation. It is an active part of life where the many psychophysiological subsystems function differently from the way they do in the wakeful part of the circadian awake–rest cycle. In addition to differences between being awake and being asleep, there also are significant differences in the psychophysiology of NREM and REM sleep.

NREM Sleep (Quiet Sleep)

During NREM sleep, most bodily functions tend to be slow, steady, and rhythmical. There is a resemblance to the relaxed, resting state while awake, but the person is not as responsive to the external environment.

As sleep moves from Stage I to Stage IV, respiration and pulse become relatively slow, regular, and rhythmical. Blood pressure and body temperature decrease, as does urinary output into the bladder. Basal skin resistance increases along with some peripheral vasodilation. Motor activity is reduced but not completely inhibited. Any eye movements that occur are slow and have a rolling character, going from side to side. Alveolar carbon dioxide increases and oxygen consumption decreases. The lowered metabolic activity is compatible with the decreased oxygen uptake. Changes in EEG are reflected in the successive stages of sleep.

NREM sleep appears to be a "retreat" into a quieter inner space, which creates its own insulating capsule that makes possible a radical decrease in the penetration of external environmental stimulation. After about 80 minutes following the onset of sleep, there seems to be an internally initiated shift back through the stages of sleep until Stage I, where the active REM phase of sleep occurs, is reached.

REM Sleep (Active Sleep)

REM sleep is also described as "active sleep" because it appears far from restful. Activation occurs in the brain and elsewhere in the central nervous system. Rapid eye movements are directly observable through the eyelids and can be recorded by an EOG of eye-muscle contractions. Paradoxically, there is an almost complete neural inhibition of striate-muscle action (so-called "sleep paralysis"). The muscles supporting the chin lose tonus, as do most of the other muscles of locomotion and action, with only the eye muscles, the anal and vesicular sphinctors, and the middle-ear contractors maintaining tonicity.

Heart rate becomes variable and accelerated. There is increased shallow breathing that also tends to be concurrent with bursts of REM. Oxygen utilization increases, and there is a decrease in blood oxygen saturation. Penile erection with the onset of REM is quite typical in the male. The pattern of EEG waves is typically that of Stage I sleep. The increase in brain temperature accompanying the rise in central nervous system activity is most evident during the bursts of REM action.

Dreaming is a dominant aspect of the REM phase of the sleep–dream cycle. Sleep laboratories have found that an ongoing dream is reported 80% or more of the time when subjects are awakened during REM sleep. Although dreaming sometimes occurs during NREM sleep, the most vivid, organized dreams are reported during REM sleep. The brain is available for constructing the dream, free from the constraints of external-world stimuli and processes involved in perceptual validation. With the internal world of sensory–cognitive stimulation available, the dream has considerable potential for meaningful content. It usually is also partly fragmented, some aspects being more or less random in the process of elaboration, diffusion, and distortion. The content may be pleasant, joyful, unpleasant, frightening, or without any special connotation. There may be some degree of correspondence between the ongoing dream content and the particular activation of body function. For example, penile erection may accompany sexual content of the dream; eye movements may be deflected upward in a dream where the individual is ascending a steep flight of stairs; and so forth. Often, however, no such apparent correspondence is evident.

The many laboratory and clinical studies of REM deprivation have amply demonstrated that mood, attitude, disposition, and behavior in the awake state may be quite adversely affected as REM deprivation accumulates. When REM deprivation ends, there is a strong effort by the individual to compensate for the REM loss through an increase in the REM proportion of sleep.

REM sleep constitutes about 20% of the total sleep time in adults, with a substantial part of that time given over to dreaming. The potential thus exists for dysphoric dream content to reflect or create stress with which the individual cannot cope as he or she might do in the awake state. This possibility gives added significance to the frequency of acute cardiac, gastrointestinal, and respiratory crises that occur during sleep, probably associated with periods of REM sleep. In some cases, it may be possible to avoid such crises through psychotherapeutic approaches that help to reduce stress and restore more restful sleep.

THEORY OF SLEEP

A clinically useful theory of sleep should provide a framework capable of encompassing at least some of the important findings of sleep research. It should also provide a rationale and direction for clinical interventions that seek to relieve the dysomnias and to transform poor sleepers into good sleepers. At present, the notion of a biphasic interactional system appears promising.

A basic postulate of this theory is that wakefulness and sleep are both active processes, one a function of an "awake generator center" and the other of a "sleep generator center." These systems actively regulate the awake–rest and the sleep–dream cycles through extensive neural connections and feedback components with the brain and central nervous system, which serve to rhythmically stimulate and inhibit their action.

Research strongly suggests that the reticular activating system, the giant neurons of the brain stem, the neurons of the dorsal raphe, and the neurons of the locus ceruleus are some of the critical components of the two generator systems. Also, the aminergic–cholinergic neurochemical system has been identified as an important dynamic controller of the interaction between the generator systems.

Another important postulate is that the awake and sleep states of the individual not only are genetically determined, but also are responsive to such ongoing events as pain, toxicity, fatigue, exercise, environmental stimulation, and intrapsychic phenomena. Sometimes the conditions of the organism act to inhibit the awake phase and to stimulate the sleep phase of the circadian cycle so that the ultradian sleep–dream cycle becomes manifest outside the typical pattern. Chemicals, relaxation experiences, and perhaps even extended involvement in fantasies may alter the conditions supporting the level of wakefulness and move the individual closer to the sleep phase of the cycle with an emergence of NREM–REM sequences. It is thought that the sleep–dream cycle remains functional throughout the 24-hour period, but that the NREM–REM sequences of sleep become manifest only when the sleep phase of the awake–rest circadian cycle gains ascendancy.

FACTORS CONTRIBUTING TO SLEEP DISORDERS

For an individual to be considered to have a sleep disorder, there must be repeated disturbances of the typical pattern of sleep, followed by an aftermath of fatigue, apathy, and other psychological malaise during the awake period.

Sleep may be beyond the reach of the individual who is agitated by fear, anxiety, and tension because of psychological stress or environmental danger. The ready shift from the awake state to the presleep state and from thence to sleep may also become difficult when there is pain, drug-induced chemical stimulation (e.g., d-amphetamine), or toxic irritability resulting in a high arousal state that overrides the sleep–dream cycle. However, even in these crisis periods, some brief episodes of sleep may occur if the crisis lasts sufficiently long. When the level of temperature, toxicity, or pain begins to be life-threatening, hypersomnolence (excessive sleep) and coma may displace wakefulness even with the coexisting high level of physiological activity. After the crisis of illness or circumstance has passed, the affected individual usually experiences a gradual re-establishment of the normal awake–rest and sleep–dream cycles, with adequate access to the onset and maintenance of sleep. For some individuals, however, the legacy of the crisis experience may be a pattern of disturbed sleep.

Disturbances in the individual's sleep pattern, such as hypersomnolence, inability to fall asleep, agitated sleep (e.g., night terrors), and sleep of insufficient duration, may be early indicators of serious psychological stress or physiological disease. Depression, suicidal impulses, psychological decompensation, and preclinical disease processes (e.g., developing sites of inflammatory reaction) may first be expressed in disturbances of the sleep pattern. In the case of psychological stress where psychological decompensation is occurring, the disturbance of sleep is apt to be self-exacerbating. The interference with sleep and deprivation of sleep can aggravate the body biochemistry, with the result that the individual experiences increased difficulty in coping with stressful situations.

Many diseases that involve high fever result in hypersomnolence lasting for days and weeks. Not only may malaria, syphilis, German measles, sleeping fever, or encephalitis profoundly affect the sleep cycle during the height of the illness, but in the young child they may leave, as a postillness consequence, some marked shifts in the circadian awake–rest cycle so that the child sleeps by day and remains wakeful during the night.

The many physiological changes that occur during sleep may aggravate existing pathology in respiration, cardiovascular action, gastrointestinal secretions, and other functions to the point of discomfort, pain, or even acute crisis. Not only may the exacerbation of existing physiological conditions (which often have a strong psychosomatic component) lead to awakening the sleeper, but the consciousness of acute discomfort may evoke anxiety about the exacerbation recurring with sleep. Angina has a well-known tendency to occur during sleep in susceptible individuals, as do episodes of elevated hypertension with associated headache, tinnitus, and related malaise. Both angina and the hypertension elevations seem to be correlated with the occurrence of REM periods. Asthma attacks seem to occur late in the night with children and about midway in the sleep cycle with adults. These episodes may be directly related to the concentrations and pressures of oxygen and carbon dioxide that occur during sleep in the blood and alveolar tissues. The increased gastric acid secretions that also occur, estimated at from 3 to 20 times those of the waking state, may result in sufficient discomfort in patients with duodenal ulcer to result in the syndrome of pain–arousal–fear–disturbed sleep.

Other conditions, such as the hypersomnolence of early pregnancy and the interrupted sleep of late pregnancy, need not indicate a sleep disorder since there may not be the accompaniment of the fatigue, apathy, and other psychological malaise in the awake phase of the circadian cycle.

Drugs, medications, and foods may significantly contribute to the occurrence of sleep disorders. Many of the most commonly used sedative–hypnotic medications (e.g., the barbiturates) diminish the amount of REM sleep time, REM dream production, and the amount of eye movements during REM. In addition, the barbiturates have a strong addictive tendency and tend to have marked morning-after "hangover effects" that add to the sluggishness of the user. There results a combined effect (REM deprivation, addiction, morning–after sluggishness, need for increased dosages) that aggravates the sleep disorder, and adds depression and other serious difficulties created by barbiturate drug habituation. Withdrawal from the use of barbiturates constitutes a health hazard by further disturbing sleep patterns and contributing to the potential danger of convulsive reactions.

Still to be definitively determined are the consequences for sleep patterns of the contraceptive pill; the mood-altering drugs that have acquired wide cultural acceptance and use; the chemical additives to food products to alter taste, appearance, and usability; the antihypertensive drugs (e.g., reserpine); and the antiappetite drugs. Such early studies as do exist suggest that many of these chemicals have significant effects upon central nervous system function and the neurochemistry of sleep, and may share in the production of sleep disorders.

Given psychological stress of various sorts and the above-listed sources of potentially provocative agents, it is not surprising that at least one-third of the general population reports sleep difficulties.

TYPES OF SLEEP DISORDERS

Dyssomnia (Insomnia)

A dyssomnia is a disturbed sleep–dream cycle followed by fatigue and psychological malaise in the waking state (depression, irritability, tension). The term "dyssomnia" more appropriately describes the disrupted sleep pattern than does "insomnia," which more strictly connotes an absence of sleep, a rare condition even on a short-term basis. Two forms of dyssomnia are described here.

For the person who has difficulty in falling asleep, there is a long delay from the time of the awake presleep state until the beginning of the NREM–REM sleep cycle. Once asleep, however, a normal NREM–REM cycle is established. The problem seems to center on the shift of state from being awake to falling asleep. There is some tendency for this type of sleep difficulty to be present in the younger adult.

In contrast is the situation where the onset time for falling asleep is within the normal range, but during the night, usually after the third NREM–REM cycle, the individual moves from REM dreaming to the awake state instead of to Stage II of NREM sleep. The individual experiences considerable difficulty in falling asleep again and feels insufficiently rested the next day. This condition is more characteristic of middle-aged adults.

Narcolepsy

Narcolepsy is characterized by the frequent and uncontrollable urge for sleep during normal waking hours. Generally the duration of sleep is brief (less than 15 minutes), although longer times have been reported. Narcolepsy is usually but not always associated with attacks of muscular tonelessness know as "cataplexy." Often, upon falling asleep, the person experiences hypnogogic hallucinations or vivid images. Persons experiencing narcolepsy are generally aware of an impending attack, and some are able to forestall the onset of sleep more successfully than others. The abrupt interruption of ongoing activities represents a serious threat if the person happens to be operating a moving vehicle or dangerous machinery. Many persons with narcolepsy, with or without cataplexy, do have accidents.

Narcolepsy can be understood as a sudden, dominating intrusion of REM-stage sleep into the waking state. REM-stage sleep is characterized not only by dreaming, but also by the paralysis of most motor-activity muscles. Thus, a narcoleptic attack may manifest a rapid plunge into a dreaming state, as well as muscle atonicity varying from slumping to limpness. It is important to note that narcolepsy is not a rare sleep disorder if one takes into account the milder forms of the disturbance.

Sleep Apnea

Sleep apnea, or the transient interruption of breathing during sleep, represents an incompatibility between the sleep state and the respiratory system. The shift of state from wakefulness to sleep generally results in an inhibition of much motor activity. In sleep apnea, this motor-inhibitory action is extended to include muscle-oriented stimuli originating from the respiratory center of the central nervous system. The intercostal muscles and the diaphragm, both essential to respiratory function, become atonic, with the result that the chest fails to expand in response to the blood concentrations of oxygen and carbon dioxide that are normally sufficient to stimulate the central nervous system's respiratory center to activate the respiratory muscles. To aggravate the respiratory problem, the throat muscles also lose their tonicity, collapse together, and further embarrass the respiratory effort.

The shift to the sleep state initiates this paralysis of the muscles essential to respiration. Oxygen deprivation and carbon dioxide accumulation have to reach a level of sufficient criticality to awaken the individual before the respiratory center becomes disinhibited, the respiratory muscle action and throat tonicity begin again, and the balance of oxygen and carbon dioxide is restored. Then the individual once again falls asleep to begin a new cycle of sleep apnea. This process sometimes repeats itself hundreds of times during the night, with perhaps one to three minutes spent in sleep, then an awake period of 3–60 seconds of restorative respiration.

The majority of individuals with sleep apnea become habituated to the multitudes of sleep–awake cycles. They forget the periods of wakening but experience a need for considerable sleep both during the night and the day. A smaller percentage, about 30%, do not habituate to the recurrent cycles and complain of dyssomnia, fatigue, and associated psychological malaise. Then there are those with sleep apnea who experience neither hypersomnia nor dyssomnia and are unaware of their problem, except that their sleeping partners may complain about their noisy sleep pattern of quiet sleep and gasping snoring that goes on throughout the night.

PSYCHOTHERAPEUTIC STRATEGIES AND HYPNOTHERAPEUTIC FACILITATIONS

Psychological treatment approaches recognize that sleep disorders are determined in part by genetic programming, in part by ongoing disturbances of physiological and psychological functioning, and in part by environmental conditions. These factors vary considerably in the extent to which they may be responsive to the effects of psychological intervention. Of course, significant physical and medical conditions need to be corrected if possible.

Psychotherapists working with people who have sleep problems share the common experience that psychological help is usually not sought early in the history of the problem. Typically, there has been encouragement by a health practitioner to use sedative–hypnotic medication, and the person continues to use such drugs even when the sleep disorder persists unchanged or has become even more disruptive. When the decision to seek psychological help is finally reached, the person may feel that the cure will be rapid and that there is no point in continuing a sustained program over time.

The goal of psychological intervention is to moderate or eliminate the disruptive internal or external conditions that interfere with the normal phase changes in the awake–rest and sleep–dream cycles. This is accomplished by (1) decreasing those conditions that stimulate the awake generator center at too high a level, thereby blocking the normal inhibitory action on this center's functioning; and (2) increasing conditions that stimulate the sleep-activating function of the sleep–dream generator center.

The planning of a comprehensive treatment program requires (1) a diagnostic study of possible organic factors involved in the disorder of sleep, including one or more nights of EEG observation (usually carried out through a medical review); (2) an assessment of sleep-related habitual behaviors and routines that sustain or even aggravate the sleep disorder; and (3) an evaluation of psychological aspects, including attitudes toward sleep and reactions to life stresses of various sorts. The client, in the role of cotherapist, plays a most important part in every phase of the treatment program: in the gathering and assessment of information, in the planning of therapeutic strategies, in the evaluation of the outcomes of the interventions, and in the designing of new approaches.

Four psychotherapeutic approaches to the treatment of sleep disorders are discussed below: alteration of sleep routines and related habits; attitude restructuring; reduction of anxiety; and facilitation of state shifts.

Alteration of Sleep Routines and Related Habits

Except for some special circumstances, disorders of sleep tend to develop over a fairly extended period of time. Poor sleep habits have the interesting position of being both a cause and a consequence of sleeping difficulties. Whereas at one time certain behaviors might not have interfered with the individual's capacity to sleep well, later they may become too stimulating. The number and intensity of these stimulating practices seem to synergize each other and to accumulate over time. The changing psychophysiological state of the client may make it increasingly difficult for him or her to isolate the stimulation from the sleep situation.

Of concern are behavioral practices that take place during the three periods in the 24-hour cycle of awake–rest that seem to have particular importance for sleep disorders: the sleep situation itself, the presleep preparation period, and the two to three hours preceding the presleep period.

A self-observation period on seven successive days is most useful for discovering those practices that need to be altered. There are many good "sleep diaries" and "sleep logs" that can be used to record events of the presleep situation, such as time of going to bed, time until onset of sleep, and the like. In addition, there are various checklists that provide behavior items relevant to sleep disorders, such as snoring, leg twitching, and the use of coffee or other drugs. The client keeps both a sleep diary and a checklist for the seven-day self-observation period and is instructed not to alter his or her usual behaviors associated with sleep, although the very act of self-observation introduces a changed awareness of the sleep situation. A uniform time for making entries in the diary and checklist, preferably in the morning soon after rising, is emphasized to assure better recall of pertinent events. The readiness of the client to invest energy in the self-observation and to integrate the record keeping into the daily activities is an indication of his or her motivation to change.

The client and therapist then analyze the self-observation data, with the goal of establishing an initial plan for altering some of the behaviors related to sleeping that might be most amenable to modification. The self-observations are also examined in terms of the client's probable circadian cycle. The initial program of change is regarded as a trial period of from one to three weeks. During this period, the client continues with the sleep diary and checklist, and may need encouragement and support in order to maintain the record keeping.

Two sleep-management problem areas appear in almost all of the seven-day self-observation baseline data: (1) *environmental-stimulation overload*—namely, ways in which the client manages to maintain a continuous influx of stimulation from the environment in the hours before sleep, in the presleep period, and in bed waiting for sleep to happen; and (2) *internal apprehension*—namely, inner tension, awareness of need to relax, inability to stop focusing upon the day just past or being preoccupied with the day ahead, and reiteration of negative thoughts about sleep and the sleep situation.

The client's record of environmental-stimulation overload may be obvious to someone else, but not to the client. Instead, the client may perceive such behavior as eating or watching television as being conducive for relaxing prior to going to sleep. The client may express considerable skepticism about the wisdom of eliminating such well-established habits. In part, this may reflect a fear that eliminating these practices might aggravate the sleep disorder. Also, these practices have been a source of some pleasure that the client may be reluctant to give up. Trust and rapport with the therapist and the need for help, however, should support the client in being willing to risk change. Together, the client and therapist decide on the changes in sleep-management practices to be attempted and the types of exercise and training to be introduced. The client also assumes responsibility for both implementing the initial program and participating in assessing its outcome.

Clinicians familiar with sleep-management practices recognize the value of certain rules or principles that help to lower the level of environmental stimulation and support the quieting of the individual. These are discussed with the client and incorporated into the treatment plan. Among these are the following:

1. *Elimination of offending substances.* Individuals vary considerably in the time needed to metabolize the stimulating effects of coffee, tea, smoking, alcohol, or other psychotropic chemicals. Even eating may be a source of arousal for some individuals. It is recommended that a systematic exploration of possibly offending substances be made with a view to determining which of these should be eliminated during the three hours prior to retiring (and, if necessary, for a period longer than that). Factors leading to the escalation or maintenance of arousal may influence the circadian rhythm long before the actual transition to falling asleep.

2. *Presleep quieting.* There is a need for a planned period of quieting before the individual begins to prepare for sleep. This is especially important when there has been considerable physical or mental activity in the latter part of the evening. The quieting period provides for a lowering of the level of arousal as well as a psychological transition to the anticipation of sleep.

3. *The bed as a place for sleeping.* For some individuals, reading, watching TV, carrying on discussions with their bed partners, reviewing the day just past, or planning the day just ahead, may be too arousing to permit sleep to ensue. In this case, these activities should be carried on outside of bed, preferably outside of the bedroom. The bed then becomes the stimulus for sleeping.

4. *Ambience of bedroom.* To keep noise, light, and other stimulating conditions to a minimun may mean eliminating pictures, statuary, work desks, and so forth from the bedroom during the therapeutic program. The bed, the coverings, and the room temperature are also factors that should be examined to maximize their comfort value. Sometimes the use of a white-noise appliance is helpful in masking intrusive sounds.

5. *Sleep intentions.* The client must learn to go to bed only when there is a felt readiness and intention to sleep. If sleep does not come after about 30 minutes, getting out of bed may be preferable to restless efforts to grasp sleep. Aggressive confrontation with the sleep situation is stimulating and counterproductive. Engaging in relaxation procedures, quieting fantasy, or meditation can be encouraged while the client lies in bed or sits in a chair until the sleep need is re-experienced.

6. *Fixed rising time.* This may be a difficult point to accept for those clients whose morning programs have flexibility and who have

accommodated themselves to late onset of sleep or difficulty in maintaining sleep by extending the sleep period well into the morning hours. However, there is much to commend the consistency of a fixed rising time for each day of the week, including the weekend, as one learns to become an adequate sleeper. The routinization of the end point of the sleep cycle tends retroactively to have a positive effect on the time of falling asleep. This incorporation of the invariable awakening time into the awake–rest pattern becomes part of positive expectations about the regularity and dependability of sleep. The expectation that falling asleep or remaining asleep will become part of one's normal experience seems to be strengthened by the consistency of morning-time arising.

7. *Curtailment of day sleep.* Sleeping periods during the day need to be curtailed until the night-time disorder has been substantially eliminated.

8. *Withdrawal of sedatives and hypnotic medications.* The planned, safe withdrawal of sedatives, hypnotic medications, and other psychotropic chemicals related to sleep is essential because of their disruptive effect upon sleep and other life adjustments.

Other changes can also help to reduce stimulation. For example, many clinicians recommend regular daily exercise, or a moderately warm bath in the presleep preparation.

Attitude Restructuring

Some attitudes toward sleep may be part of the individual's sleep problem. For example, the attitude that links sleep with death may be a source of anxiety, fear, and active avoidance of the sleep situation. The cross-cultural prevalence of this attitude suggests that it may be a part of the general human experience of growing up, of passing through early childhood when so much of sleep time is spent in REM-stage dreaming sleep. The frequency of night terrors, reluctance to sleep in the dark, and other sleep problems of that age period may in part reflect the child's limited capacity to differentiate among sleep–dream experiences, awake-fantasy experiences, and reality. Important here are cognitive problems of reality testing that are related to early stages in the development of critical thinking.

A second childhood experience that may reinforce the sleep–death association is the custom of presleep prayers (such as "Now I Lay Me Down to Sleep") that emphasize the association between sleep and death. The hundreds of repetitions of such prayers, night after night, may form a strong psycholinguistic and emotional bond between these two states until they merge into a single concept.

In the course of daily living, almost everyone observes someone else asleep. The body posture of the sleeper, the loss of facial expression, the immobility, and the appearance of the sleeper as having withdrawn from contact with the world into an inner space inaccessible to the observer may all contribute their share to reinforcing the death–sleep, sleep–death association. Finally, there are probably close linkages between the feeling that sleep represents a loss of control by the individual over both the self and the environment and the attitude toward sleep as partial death.

Communication of accurate information about the nature of sleep is an early therapeutic procedure to counterbalance the distorted perception of sleep represented in the sleep–death association. Such communication stresses the basic ideas that sleep is a natural, genetically programmed phenomenon; that sleep difficulties have to be learned; and therefore that it is quite possible to learn how to re-establish conditions for restoring normal and refreshing sleep.

How people come to link sleep and death on the basis of early experiences can then be discussed in order to help the client understand that such associations are common and well known and that they represent learning processes rather than weird obsessions. The participation of the client in the discussion helps the client to explore his or her own early memories about related events.

In utilizing hypnosis for further exploration, the client needs training in how to enter the trance state of consciousness and invite mental images and fantasies. With these skills, the client can then be encouraged to experience the dual roles of observer and participant in exploring recollections that may have linked sleep with death. (See Chapter 7, "Dissociation.")

As observer, the client remains in the present time frame in active contact with the psychotherapist, while as participant, the client also experiences the past through fantasy or mental imagery. The observer is encouraged to communicate with the experiencing participant, to explain to the participant how this misunderstanding about sleep has occurred, and to give the participant as much of an explanation as that self is able to assimilate. When religious practices or beliefs become involved, the observer helps the participant to understand that a concrete interpretation of a prayer or ritual is apt to be made by a child and might become frightening. The therapist can help the observer share other examples, as when a parent's adoring statement, "You are so sweet I could eat you up," might become nightmarish to the literal-minded child, even though its loving intent is absolutely understood by the adult. The observing self works with the participating self to transform frightening, literal associations with sleep to their more reassuring symbolic meanings. It may be necessary for the client, in the two coexisting roles of observer and participant, to "relive" a given fantasy more than once before ideo-motor signaling (see pp. 29–31) would indicate that the negative connotations have been desensitized or dissolved. Similar exploration of other negative episodes and settings related to the sleep problem may be indicated.

The attitude-restructuring process may also be facilitated by using trance to associate sleep with pleasant experiences such as rest, recuperation, and dream fun. As an important by-product, the training in shifting from the awake state to the trance state in the course of the desensitization–restructuring process may also be useful in learning how to shift from the awake to the asleep state.

A very different type of attitude involves beliefs held by the person about his or her own sleep experiences. Actually, the beliefs themselves constitute the sleep problem. The person may perceive himself or herself as a chronic dyssomniac who has difficulties with almost every aspect of sleeping: the onset of sleep, the maintenance of sleep, and the duration of sleep. The client's self-image, sincerely believed, is that of being a "nonsleeper." Sleep is seen as forever elusive; each night is remembered as a waking vigil with brief interruptions of drowsiness. Not only is the person preoccupied with problems of sleep, but there also may be a readiness to attribute responsibility for discrepancies between personal potential and actual achievement to the burden of being chronically beset with insomnia.

In many cases, EEG night-time records reveal a quite adequate night sleep pattern in all respects, with the exception of perhaps one to four brief awakenings, followed by a fairly rapid return to sleep. When night sleep and daytime naps are combined, most norms of an adequate amount of sleep would be met. However, when such a client is asked to maintain a sleep log and to describe his or her sleep history, the reported experiences seem compatible with those of nonsleepers, except that there does not seem to be an accumulation of fatigue and psychological malaise. Because the person suffers no ill effects other than believing that he or she is unable to sleep, the dyssomnia may be characterized as a pseudoproblem.

Yet the nonsleeper self-perception is quite real. It is as if the person experiences an active and almost immediate retrograde amnesia for each of the night's sleep episodes and a vivid memory of each of the awake times. The brief awake times then merge together and are extended in time, while the actual sleep times between the awake periods are confabulated into a conviction of having been almost continuously awake.

For many clients, the evidence of the EEG records, together with a focus on their general state of health and on the effectiveness of their daily life activities, makes possible a shift in self-image from "nonsleeper" to "adequate sleeper." Hypnotherapeutic explorations of possible secondary gains that may be associated with the idea of being a nonsleeper can be productive in helping such a client to accept the reinterpretation of sleep competence and to search for alternate ways of achieving goals that were previously regarded as being blocked by chronic dyssomnia.

Reduction of Anxiety: Example of Sleep Suggestions during Relaxation

Sleep may be disrupted because the situation of going to sleep generates anxiety in the individual, or because there is an ongoing state of anxiety concerning other life events that carries over to the sleep situation. In either case, the existence of anxiety means that the individual has an additional quantum of vigilance–arousal impinging on the central nervous system that may interfere with the cyclical appearance of the sleep phase of the awake–rest cycle.

Anxiety generated by the sleep situation itself is almost always associated with attitudes toward sleep—with beliefs that link sleep with death or other threatening possibilities. The preceding discussion on attitude restructuring deals with psychotherapeutic interventions that seek to reduce or eliminate this anxiety-inducing capacity of the sleep situation. There are occasions, of course, when anxiety or fear about going to sleep may be completely appropriate to the realities of

270 III. Special Clinical Problems

a dangerous environmental situation. In such circumstances, delays in the onset of sleep and the maintenance of a light, vigilant, easily aroused sleep are adaptive to the existing threat. Such a disruption of the normal sleep pattern is not a sleep disorder; it becomes such only when the threat has long since passed but the disruption of the sleep pattern continues.

Ongoing difficulties in the waking life of an individual may generate varying degrees of anxiety. When this anxiety persists at a relatively high level into the presleep period, there is maintained a continuing stimulation of the awake generator center that may counterbalance the usual inhibitory action of the sleep generator, with a consequent disturbance in the normal emergence, maintenance, and duration of sleep. This situation presents two separate but closely related therapeutic problems: (1) the need to deal with and if possible resolve these life stresses that are generating excessive anxiety, and (2) the need to reduce the arousal level in the presleep period resulting from the anxiety reaction in order to permit the sleep generator's effects to gain ascendancy.

The client's readiness to support the proposition that better sleep will provide more energy to cope with daytime problems facilitates acceptance of the idea that life-stress anxiety can be confined and need not spill over to interfere with drifting off to sleep. Thus, an early psychotherapeutic priority in such situations is to help the client accept the possibility that presleep anxiety can be reduced. The techniques of ideomotor inquiry, such as the use of the Chevreul pendulum, can be helpful in evaluating the readiness of the client to accept this proposition and, if so, to move on toward a containment of that anxiety.

The client in the following example had had training in the use of breathing exercises and progressive relaxation as well as in the use of the Chevreul pendulum.

THERAPIST: [To the client in the waking state:] Let's ask the pendulum if the inner part of your mind is ready to improve the quality of your sleep so that you may have more energy and strength to give to your daytime problems. [The pendulum action is slow to start. The first clear movement is clockwise, an "I don't know" response. It then changes over into a definite, strong "yes."] The pendulum began with a weak "I don't know" response and then shifted over into a strong, definite "yes" that persisted. This is very typical when someone is uncertain of how they will make out with something new that they know they want but haven't tried as yet. However, the strong "yes" must mean that the inner part of your mind is pretty sure of what it wants.

Let's ask the inner part of your mind if it is okay for us to take the first steps toward better sleep right now. [The pendulum response is a quick "yes."] That answer is certainly clear enough. Last week you practiced the muscle-tensing and the muscle-relaxing exercises . . . Go through the sequence on your own . . . [The client repeats the progressive-relaxation exercise that had been learned the previous week.]

Good . . . We can proceed to the breathing exercise that helped you to make your relaxation so much better . . . Follow the air that you are breathing in from the outside. Feel it pass through your nose, into your mouth and throat, and down into your lungs, filling them up with the fresh air down to the smallest subdivision and feel your chest expand. Now follow the air out . . . Feel your lungs relax and the chest muscles let go as the air flows upward through your throat, into your mouth, moving over your tongue and through your lips, carrying out the used air.

Let your total relaxation expand with each movement of the air into your lungs and out of them . . . As you feel and hear and taste the airflow, let yourself drift into your own quiet inner space . . . peaceful . . . away from the pressures of the daytime . . . free from having to do anything about the problems of the daytime . . . Know that these problems can wait for tomorrow . . . Know that "the morning is wiser than the evening" . . . that you can wait until tomorrow to think about these problems . . . You are not forgetting about these problems . . . You can think about them tomorrow . . . Now the inner part of your mind is guiding you into this quiet, special, secure inner space of your own where sleep can enter when you are ready for it to refresh your body and mind . . . When you are in this special place, let the index finger of your right hand signal. . . . [The client signals.]

Very good . . . Let your inner mind do whatever is right for you to make this special inner place of yours restful, quiet, secure . . . You can let your own image of sleep enter this inner place of yours whenever you are ready to make it welcome . . . to become part of the quiet . . . helping to release any tensions that might possibly still be present . . . letting go . . . enjoying the release . . . enjoying the presence of sleep in your quiet security. . . .

In your own home . . . when you are at rest in your special inner space . . . you can let your image of sleep extend to the full inner space . . . There is nothing you have to do . . . It is the natural flow of living . . . With each breath you take, your body will use the sleep to restore its strength and well-being until your full need for sleep is complete . . . Then . . . when your sleep need is fulfilled . . . each breath will bring you comfortably and refreshed to becoming awake . . . anticipating the day ahead. . . .

In a few moments I shall count from ONE to FIVE . . . With each count, you can permit as much inner subjective time to pass as you may desire to make the transition to the here and now welcome and pleasant. After you are in the here and now . . . with the consent of the inner part of your mind . . . you can repeat the total exercise in every detail so that it becomes more and more part of your own capability . . . Your right index finger just gave the "yes" signal, so it will be in order for you to repeat the exercise . . . I will be here to help guide you should you need any guiding. . . .

ONE . . . leaving this quiet restful inner space with the full knowledge that it is there for your use whenever desired . . . TWO . . . eyelids feeling the flutter coming into them as they prepare to open . . . THREE . . . eyes opening fully, quietly, absorbing the here and now . . . FOUR . . . the relaxation and the peacefulness remaining with you . . . FIVE . . . fully into the here and now. . . .

Notice that while the client was being guided toward becoming relaxed and peaceful, the therapist also gave the reassurance that there was a better time to deal with problems, that "the morning is wiser than the evening." This helped the client bind off the concerns of the day for the time being—concerns that the client knew would not simply disappear, and on the contrary, required some form of resolution.

There are many variations in the ways in which hypnotic trance can be used to reduce anxiety. As seen in the example above, the particular sequence of a progressive-relaxation exercise (muscle tensing–relaxing), then the yoga-like focus upon the flow of life-giving air into and out of the lungs, and finally the movement into the security of the inner space of mind and self where sleep may enter, constitutes a triad of clinically useful experiences. For the individual with disturbed sleep because of daytime anxiety, the reduction in the arousal level, together with the suggestion that problems can be deferred for more effective daytime handling, permits the sleep generator center to function more normally.

Practice at home is a key to the acquisition of skill in segregating daytime anxiety from the sleep situation and in preparing the self for a more comfortable and controlled transition into the sleep state. The exercises for the night-time control of anxiety also have the broader utility of being useful in the treatment of daytime stresses as well, whatever the psychotherapeutic approach may be.

Facilitation of State Shifts: Example of Dissociation

As mentioned earlier, wakefulness and sleep are manifestations of a biphasic interactional system consisting of an awake generator center and a sleep generator center, which function to create two dynamic, interacting, genetically based cycles—namely, the awake–rest circadian cycle and the sleep–dream ultradian cycle. This system operates quite regularly and smoothly with minor variations unless ongoing internal or external events disrupt the sequence. The system is most vulnerable to disruption at the points of transition from one state or phase to another. Thus, most sleep disorders tend to occur in the transition zone of the circadian awake–rest cycle, when one is moving from wakefulness to sleep, and in the transition zone of the sleep–dream cycle, when REM-stage sleep is ready to deepen into NREM sleep.

Some problems related to the onset and maintenance of sleep are less related to anxiety than to difficulty in shifting from one state of consciousness or being to another. Difficulty in shifting may be a more general problem, however, than just a problem in the sleep situation. It may also be a problem in shifting from work to play, from displeasure to contentment, from being close to someone to letting go, and so forth. If the hypothesis of difficulty in shifting from one state to another is valid, then psychotherapeutic interventions that seek to provide the client with "transitional" techniques to facilitate such shifting could be helpful.

Dissociation techniques utilizing hypnosis can be useful in easing the transition between the awake state and the asleep state as well as in maintaining sleep. The client who has already learned how to self-induce trance can be instructed to use eye fixation, hand levitation, or some other procedure requiring motoric action in order to focus attention upon muscle tonus before proceeding to relaxation. Such motoric involvement is in itself a change-of-state experience, followed by another shift to the state of relaxation.

The following demonstration shows how one client was guided to experience creative dissociation following trance induction:

THERAPIST: [After self-induction of trance by the client.] Very good . . . Let your physical self continue with its relaxation. What would be the most pleasing physical comfort that you could imagine?

CLIENT: What I would like would be a fantastic foam-rubber mattress that would wrap around my body and conform to me like a glove. It would be so soft that I would feel absolutely no pressure beneath me, yet so firm in its support that it would be massaging every inch of skin on my back.

T: What a wonderful mattress . . . Your physical self should find such a foam-rubber rest totally comfortable . . . Let me know by a finger signal when you see yourself resting comfortably . . . [The client raises the right index finger.] Check yourself over to be sure that you are absolutely comfortable: that your arms, legs, back, and every part of you is completely relaxed . . . Describe yourself. . . .

C: [Voice is very soft and low.] I see myself resting very comfortably, and the foam rubber is hugging me all around just like a glove. . . .

T: Any time that your physical self needs to change position, it can do so with ease . . . since that part of you is resting so comfortably . . . [The therapist introduces the possibility of dissociation:] Let's ask your fingers if it would be okay to take off and explore your own inner space of images, thoughts, and feelings while your physical self continues to rest on the foam-rubber mattress. [The client signals "yes."] Should your physical self move over into sleep while you are in your inner space, or should you begin to feel sleepy, you can easily merge back with your physical self and continue what you were doing. . . .

You may want to use your inner space to find a place of total quiet or relaxation, or you might want to revisit a time or event of special importance that was a good experience for yourself. You can also use your inner space to have a play or TV show that would help you understand yourself . . . or a sheer fun trip . . . Signal with your right index finger when your inner mind has entered its inner space

. . . Good, you can feel free to share or not to share what is going on . . .

[The client describes an emotional reunion with family members and then talks about nostalgically meeting old friends. The therapist acknowledges the reported experiences as the client shares them, and then returns to the matter of sleep:]

T: What is your favorite way of placing your physical self in getting ready for sleep?

C: I turn on my right side . . . and my arm is around my pillow and my head is on the pillow . . . My left hand is usually across my chest . . . My legs are partly drawn up, the left one a little ahead of the right one. . . .

T: Would you like to check back on your physical self and arrange yourself in that typical position? [The client signals "yes."] You can blend back into yourself at any time and continue with your family reunion . . . Should you fall asleep, the merging will occur automatically and immediately . . . When you are relaxing at home, you will be passing over into sleep at some time. However, while your mind is active, your body will be resting, relaxing, and sleeping . . . You can instruct yourself to awake in the morning after you have had a good night's rest feeling rested and relaxed . . .

Now, give yourself the signal to return to the here and now. . . .

Dissociation techniques also have special psychotherapeutic relevance for the treatment of many sleep-maintenance dyssomnias. The first experience of arousal from sleep, with difficulty falling asleep again, usually does not cause much concern in the person. However, when these arousals begin to occur more frequently and fatigue and irritability are experienced the next day, then the person becomes apprehensive about the awakenings. The mobilization of anxiety aggravates the problem by heightening the general level of arousal and extending the awake period.

Just as in the case of the client having difficulty with the onset of sleep, the client who has difficulty maintaining sleep is given training in the induction of trance, practice with progressive relaxation, and then skill in the use of a dissociation procedure. The aim of the training is to move rapidly from the decision to enter into trance to involvement in the dissociation process. Then, when the client becomes aware of no longer being asleep, he or she can learn immediately to give the self the cue to shift into hypnotic trance and the dissociation procedure. The body is still at rest, having been involved only moments before in the "sleep paralysis" of REM-stage sleep. Instead of mobilizing anxiety, the trance state contains the arousal level at a substantially lower level and directs the mental activity into the self-accepting fantasy realm. The individual continues in a state of rest and relaxation during the awake period until sleep is re-established.

The client, as cotherapist, comes to share in the understanding of why some old habits need changing, why new patterns of sleep management need to be acquired, and why recurrences of sleep disturbance occasionally are part of the mastery of new coping skills. The client also learns how to make use of quieting exercises, trance induction, imagery evocation, dissociation, and other hypnosis procedures as aids in that mastery. Anxiety and stress stemming from old and contemporaneous life experiences may also need psychotherapeutic attention in order to optimize the restorative function of sleep. Here, too, hypnosis may be incorporated into the psychotherapy. In most cases, the client is able ultimately to move from the role of cotherapist to that of self-therapist in the management of sleep and related problems.

Crisis Hypnotherapy

The words "crisis" and "critical" derive from the Greek root meaning "decision" or "turning point." Physicians have long designated that particular moment in the course of a patient's illness when there seems to be a turning point for the better or worse as the "crisis." A "critical" condition may arise because a paroxysmal onset of pain or disordered function threatens the integrity of the individual. In the literary and psychological realms, the term "crisis" has been used to describe those emotionally significant events that have resulted in, or have had the potential for creating, radical change in an individual's status. The notion of crisis is also descriptively relevant to distressed interpersonal relationships when radical changes seem imminent.

Two broad categories of crisis situations should be distinguished because of their differential implications for therapy: namely, the crisis of catastrophic onset and of more slowly developing onset.

CATASTROPHIC CRISIS

The catastrophic type of crisis is sudden in onset. Typically, there is a massive, destructive assault upon the integrity of the physical and psychological person. The crisis can be precipitated by physical trauma or by psychological difficulties. In both instances, body–mind interdependency provides the basis for the potential usefulness of hypnotherapeutic approaches, even when the person is unconscious.

Note: This chapter is based on the author's presidential address to the Division of Psychological Hypnosis of the American Psychological Association, at the annual APA convention, New Orleans, Louisiana, 1974.

Example of Traumatic Accident

The catastrophic-onset crisis is most vividly illustrated by the traumatic accident—the situation where, in a matter of seconds, an individual is transformed from a reasonably healthy, well-functioning, socially oriented person into someone struggling to survive at the most basic biological level. The body shock is most often expressed via marked alterations of consciousness, disturbances in orientation, fear, and seriously disrupted physiological functioning. Although an external accident is the most frequent basis for such trauma, the same impact may also be experienced from an internal cerebrovascular or cardiovascular accident.

Clinical evidence indicates that critically injured persons are highly accessible to suggestions, both constructive and destructive. That is why it is important to train ambulance attendants in how to communicate to seriously injured persons from the moment of initial contact at the scene of an accident until arrival at the hospital. Supportive suggestions should be offered in a continuing flow, whether or not the person appears conscious. The hypnotherapeutic character of these suggestive messages is apparent from the following transcript:

THERAPIST: You are in good hands now. You will be at the hospital shortly. Everything there is being made ready to help you. Let your muscles relax, let your mind begin to feel more secure and quiet . . . Wherever this may be needed, let your blood vessels adjust to keep the blood circulating inside your blood vessels and to seal off leaks if they occur . . . Wherever your skin is tight and tense, let it relax and permit the body's healing processes begin to work . . . As you listen to my voice, you will find yourself gradually becoming calmer . . . Your breath will move in and out of your chest more freely and more regularly . . . Your body has already begun to mobilize its healing powers and started to repair your hurt . . . Everything that can be done to help you right here is now being done. Soon you will be at the hospital. The medical team has been told that you are on your way in. The team will take over with the hospital's resources to help you. . . .

The intent of the communication is always to help the injured person to become less fearful, to feel more secure and relaxed, and to engage the healing resources of the body at that moment.

Example of Burn Wounds

It seems reasonable to hypothesize that there is a critical period in the normal mobilization of the body's defenses after a burn where some degree of control of the skin's reaction by the injured person is possible, so that enough but not too much reddening of the skin, exudate formation, and cellular reaction can take place. It is likely that the diminution of fear and anxiety plays a significant role in the body's complex defense system against injury. The hypnotic induction at a critical moment, with the suggestion of coolness and the reassuring assertion that healing is already actively under way, can be expected to be helpful and clearly cannot be harmful. The following case was reported by a physician with an active medical practice specializing in industrial emergencies.

B. B. was burned while lighting a furnace without realizing that the gas was on. He sustained first-degree burns on his entire face except for two small patches of skin. He was taken to the emergency clinic where the physician went through a rapid hypnosis procedure and then suggested coolness of the skin. As the suggestions continued, the redness of the skin faded somewhat, and the puffiness of the eyelids decreased. It was then suggested that B. B. would find the sensations coming from his face quite tolerable, and that the process of healing had already begun. By the end of the first postburn day, B. B. was able to open his eyelids—a response that usually requires several posttrauma days with the extent of burn that he had sustained. He reported that he had made use only of some mild analgesic, and none of the Darvon available to him. By the fourth postburn day, despite the physician's admonition not to enter high-heat areas, B. B. had returned to work and made occasional entries into the heat area. He shaved on the fifth day, and was discharged as sufficiently healed on the ninth postburn day.

Severe burn wounds are an example of a catastrophic event with considerable pain occurring not only initially, but during much of the healing process. Hypnotherapists have demonstrated that hypnosis can be used to great advantage in the management of protracted difficult problems such as are involved in dressing changes, transplants of skin, and the management of adequate nutrition. A detailed example of the use of dissociation during hypnotic trance to help the person relieve the distress of burn-dressing changes is presented in Chapter 7 (pp. 113–117).

Example of Attempted Suicide

The following case history illustrates a catastrophic crisis precipated by psychological difficulties:

Mrs. A. B. had been seen in psychotherapy for several months, with only small progress in the resolution of her depression. She was a 45-year-old mother of three children whose youngest son had been killed in a motor accident three years earlier while on a trip with his grandmother. Mrs. A. B., who had encouraged the child to go on the trip, felt herself directly responsible for his death. She had been in grief since the accident, had closed off her son's room, and did not allow anyone to enter or anything to be disturbed. She had also begun to drink heavily.

On this particular day, she was admitted into the emergency room shortly after midnight in a deep coma, with failing respiration and lowering of other vital signs. She had ingested an unknown quantity of barbiturates and was in a deep critical state. Her husband was certain that not more than 45 minutes had elapsed since A. B. went up to her bedroom. Stomach lavage was immediately instituted by the emergency-room physician; her internist and her psychotherapist arrived within less than 10 minutes after receiving the emergency-room call. They began administering artificial respiration, alternating in shifts, for the next six hours. Sustaining procedures such as nasal oxygen and intravenous fluids were also instituted.

Almost immediately upon contact with A. B., the therapist began to talk to her even though she was in deep coma, had a loss of corneal reflexes, and was unable to maintain her own respiration:

THERAPIST: The worst is over. You have fully discharged whatever guilt you might still have felt about D.'s death. Now you are going to be reborn into life for yourself, for your children, and for your husband . . . With each breath that passes through your lungs, your body will cleanse out the chemicals you took to gain relief from your long grief . . . As the chemicals clear out, and your own body processes return to health, you will feel your physical and emotional health returning. You will experience yourself coming back into life . . . The grieving is finished . . . You will always be able to recall the joyous moments of D.'s life . . . Soon you will begin to feel a lightness and brightness inside of yourself as you move along in your rebirth and return to life . . . Let every part of your body, your mind, your spirit, move you along this pathway to living with yourself, your family, and your friends. With each breath passing through your lungs, feel yourself becoming whole again. . . .

With very little variation, the suggestions were continued for the whole period of the assisted respiration. After six hours, Mrs. A. B. took over control of her own respiration. Cardiac function was regular and strong, and she was transferred to the intensive care unit. Twelve hours after admission, the nurse called the therapist to say that Mrs. A. B. was awake and very much wanted to see him.

Mrs. A. B. was alert, sitting up, and smiling. She seemed calm. She apologized for all the trouble and worry she had caused her husband and her therapist, feeling that the suicide attempt was such a foolish thing to do—especially since she now felt that life was so precious. She added that she felt as if she was "reborn," as if a load had been taken off her back, and as if something was finally finished. She vaguely remembered a very bright light beckoning her from afar, and a voice that faded in and out but seemed to be reaching inside of her, taking out some painful things that were preventing her from coming together again. She could not identify whose voice it was, but she knew and trusted the voice. She said that she had swallowed about 40 or more 1½-grain phenobarbital pills that she had deliberately collected from several physicians. Fortunately, she had not drunk alcohol that evening.

Mrs. A. B. felt well enough by evening to want to leave the hospital. She was released the following day, without any of the all-too-frequent respiratory complications following massive overdose of barbiturates. During the following weeks, she made rapid progress in her psychotherapy. The alcoholism was a completely settled issue. Mrs. A. B. has maintained her improvement, save for two or three minor episodes of depression, for many years since the suicide attempt; she has managed a real-estate business and involved herself actively with her adolescent and postadolescent children.

The therapist's intervention was active, directive, and supportive, with full use being made of hypnotherapeutic suggestions. A deeply felt responsibility for the well-being of Mrs. A. B. was evident. It was clear that at the time of the suicide crisis she was capable of very limited responsiveness, participation, and self-direction. The therapist undertook the task of helping the client to move toward a more active functioning.

The catastrophic type of crisis onset usually severely impairs the person's capacity for initiative and self-direction. The shock of the trauma, the physical helplessness, and the psychological disarray are part of what constitute the crisis. In this situation, the therapist accepts the fully dependent state of the person. Therapeutic activity is unidirectional, with almost no feedback from the person to guide the therapeutic suggestions. The therapist recognizes the altered state of consciousness of the person and the person's very limited potential for overt response at the time of the crisis. Yet it is important to communicate messages that the traumatized person can begin to absorb whenever sufficient attention capability emerges at whatever level of psychological functioning.

The therapist proceeds on the basis that some of the conditions associated with the hypnotic state are present; however, because of the incapacity of the person to participate in a comanagement role, a directive type of suggestion is considered most appropriate. On a very basic level, the assumption that it is possible to achieve hypnotherapeutic rapport enables the therapist to continue relating to the individual as a *person* over a fairly extended period of time with practically no interacting social relationship or feedback.

THE DEVELOPING CRISIS: EXAMPLE OF THREATENED SUICIDE

The second category of crisis referred to above is the "developing crisis." In this type of crisis, the escalating emotional stress threatens the individual's sense of integrity and control as a functioning person. Yet at least a modest capacity to become actively engaged in the therapeutic process remains. It is this capacity that makes possible, and even requires, a very different type of hypnotherapeutic intervention from that used in catastrophic crisis.

Hypnotherapeutic intervention in a developing crisis situation aims at maintaining or extending the self-directive and decision-making capabilities of the client. It strives to moderate the disruptive effects of the mounting emotional complexities and to assist the client in finding a way to effect helpful changes in himself or herself and the situation. The individual may or may not be in therapy at the time of the crisis. The psychotherapist, whatever his or her theoretical framework and values may be, is obliged to assume a moderately active role in the crisis intervention, but only to provide sufficient support to enable the client to move responsibly toward a resolution of the crisis based upon the client's needs and capabilities.

Two hypnotic strategies have significant value when a situation of crisis proportions is developing. The first is aimed at lowering the emotionally disruptive aspects of the crisis through physical and psychological relaxation, utilizing the client's own capabilities rather than medication. The decision of the client to accept relaxation procedures indicates that the wish and hope for improvement remain as a viable life force to be mobilized. Through involving the client in decision making, the need of the client to regain a sense of control is also supported. The relaxation procedures themselves help the client to become less anxious and partially disengaged from the crisis situation, thereby creating conditions favorable for the consideration of alternative ways of viewing and dealing with the crisis situation.

The second hypnotherapeutic strategy draws upon the heightened vividness of fantasy, imagination, and memory in the altered state of consciousness called hypnosis. The therapist may make use of a wide range of hypnotherapeutic possibilities, including guided imagery, projective techniques, hypnodrama, and other approaches that fit with the psychotherapeutic work of resolving some of the crisis aspects of the situation. The choice of the given hypnotherapeutic intervention is, of course, dependent upon the psychotherapeutic orientation of the particular therapist and the specifics of the client's crisis.

D. S. was a 38-year-old physicist whose depression, self-devaluation, and work difficulties had become markedly aggravated by his wife's decision to move into a separate apartment. He began to make frequent references to the futility of life, his loss of appetite, the difficulties in getting to his job in the morning, and his need for alcohol in order to get to sleep at night. The growing potential for a suicidal move was recognized by both the therapist and the client. At one therapy session, there seemed to be a qualitatively different tone to the client's depression; the therapist interpreted this as a sharp movement toward a decision to commit suicide.

The therapist proposed that D. actively explore the dimensions of taking his own life while in hypnosis. D. was experienced in utilizing hypnotic trance in therapy and agreed to the proposal. He was able to relax sufficiently, and then, while in trance, was asked to place himself "in trauma." With the guidance of the therapist, he chose and described his own method of self-destruction, prepared a letter to his wife that was filled with bitter accusations, and fantasized the carrying out of his own death. He was then asked to describe in detail the discovery of his body; the reactions of his wife, family, and friends; and the burial procedure. He was also asked to move time forward—to describe his wife's life for a year after his death, to look at his successor in his job, and to see some of his friends. He was then asked to describe his own remains at the end of the year. Moments of intense grief accompanied the burial and the postburial imagery. This suicide fantasy was re-experienced three times from beginning to end. The therapist then asked the client if he wanted to make any changes in any part of the scenario, to which D. responded that he did not wish to make a single change.

During the posthypnotic review of the suicide, there was a considerable amount of quiet crying. At the end of the session, D. expressed a sense of great relief, saying that he felt himself freed from the pressure toward suicide as the only resolution of his difficulties. While he would not rule out the continued possibility of suicide, he now felt that he was not being pushed and pulled toward suicide; suicide instead felt like a distant unreality. During the next few therapy sessions, the suicide solution became less and less attractive, the depressed feelings were considerably lightened, and the client became much more actively oriented toward considering alternative life choices.

Whether a situation can best be described as one that is developing into a crisis or one that is in fact catastrophic is not always obvious. When the person is unconscious, with life itself being threatened, then the situation is clear. But what if the person is conscious, but so decompensated and fragmented that the ability to concentrate is highly limited or ideation is bizarre? Ultimately it must be the considered judgment of the therapist as to whether hypnotherapy is feasible or even the medium of choice. Sometimes the decision will be that a protective environment, such as hospitalization, is needed before psychotherapy can be considered. Sometimes drug therapy will be regarded as a prerequisite to the possibility of successful psychotherapeutic intervention.

This last chapter has extended the range of hypnotherapeutic applications to situations that require a more or less directive approach. Even in emergency situations, however, respect for the person's struggle and potential for growth should remain intact and should guide the behavior of the therapist, both in relating to the client and in arriving at a decision concerning the appropriateness of psychotherapy or hypnotherapy.

The preceding chapters have dealt with the place of hypnotherapy in psychotherapy, hypnotherapeutic techniques, and application to a diversity of clinical problems. The reader will have become aware of the extent to which the discussion and demonstrations are based upon my beliefs concerning the nature of human development and potential for change. Psychotherapists are encouraged to make use of those concepts and procedures that they can support, to extend them in productive ways, and to transform others in accordance with their own belief systems.

Index